# THE COMPLETE BEGINNERS GUIDE TO DIET AND EXERCISE FOR SENIORS

A Step-By-Step Plan to Boost Health, Build Strength and Flexibility, Improve Balance and Mental Focus to Achieve an Active Life

## ALEX SILVER

© Copyright Alex Silver 2024 - **All rights reserved.**

The content within this book may not be reproduced, duplicated or transmitted without direct written permission from the author or the publisher.

Under no circumstances will any blame or legal responsibility be held against the publisher, or author, for any damages, reparation, or monetary loss due to the information contained within this book. Either directly or indirectly. You are responsible for your own choices, actions, and results.

**Legal Notice:**

This book is copyright protected. This book is only for personal use. You cannot amend, distribute, sell, use, quote or paraphrase any part, of the content within this book, without the consent of the author or publisher.

**Disclaimer Notice:**

Please note the information contained within this document is for educational and entertainment purposes only. All effort has been expended to present accurate, up-to-date, and reliable, complete information. No warranties of any kind are declared or implied. Readers acknowledge that the author is not engaging in the rendering of legal, financial, medical or professional advice. The content within this book has been derived from various sources. Please consult a licensed professional before attempting any techniques outlined in this book.

By reading this document, the reader agrees that under no circumstances is the author responsible for any losses, direct or indirect, which are incurred as a result of the use of the information contained within this document, including, but not limited to, — errors, omissions, or inaccuracies.

## Medical Disclaimer

The information provided in this book is for educational and informational purposes only and is not intended as medical advice. The content is not a substitute for professional medical diagnosis, advice, or treatment. Always seek the guidance of a qualified healthcare professional before making changes to your diet, exercise routine, or health practices.

The author and publisher are not medical professionals and make no representations or warranties concerning the accuracy, applicability, or completeness of the content. The recommendations in this book may not be suitable for everyone, and individual results may vary.

By using this book, you acknowledge and agree that the author and publisher are not responsible for any adverse effects, injuries, or outcomes that may occur from implementing the information or recommendations provided. If you have or suspect that you have a medical condition, consult with a healthcare provider before taking any action based on this book.

## Table of Contents

Introduction — 9

1. THE FOUNDATION OF HEALTH: UNDERSTANDING DIET AND EXERCISE FOR SENIORS — 13
   1.1 Why Diet Comes First: The Foundation of Health — 14
   1.2 Metabolic Health: The Key to Effective Exercise — 15
   1.3 The Role of Nutrition in Aging Well — 17
   1.4 Overcoming Common Diet and Exercise Myths — 20
   1.5 Setting Realistic and Achievable Health Goals — 23

2. UNCONVENTIONAL DIETS: EXPLORING KETO, CARNIVORE, AND PALEO — 27
   2.1 The Keto Diet: High Fat, Low Carb for Seniors — 27
   2.2 Carnivore Diet: Meat-Centric Nutrition — 30
   2.3 Paleo Diet: Eating Like Our Ancestors — 33
   2.4 Comparing the Diets: Which One is Right for You? — 35
   2.5 Transitioning to a New Diet: Tips and Tricks — 38

3. DOCTOR-APPROVED DIETS: INSIGHTS FROM THE EXPERTS — 41
   3.1 Dr. Shawn Baker – Coined the Phrase "Carnivore Diet" — 41
   3.2 Dr. Ken Berry on the Keto/Carnivore Diet — 45
   3.3 Dr. Eric Westman's Approach to Low-Carb Living — 48
   3.4 Dr. Annette Bosworth's Insights on Metabolic Health — 50
   3.5 Dr. Anthony Chaffee's Nutritional Wisdom — 53

4. PRACTICAL MEAL PLANNING: MAKING DIET WORK FOR YOU — 57
   4.1 Meal Planning Template and Practical Tips — 58
   4.2 Nutrient-Dense Foods for Seniors — 60
   4.3 Easy and Delicious Keto Recipes — 62

| | |
|---|---|
| 4.4 Simple Carnivore Meals | 65 |
| 4.5 Paleo-Friendly Dishes | 68 |

### 5. STARTING AN EXERCISE ROUTINE: GETTING MOVING SAFELY — 73

| | |
|---|---|
| 5.1 Assessing Your Current Fitness Level | 73 |
| 5.2 Warm-Up and Cool-Down Exercises | 76 |
| 5.3 Walking for Health: The Easiest Exercise | 78 |
| 5.4 Chair Exercises: Staying Active with Limited Mobility | 80 |
| 5.5 Flexibility and Stretching: Preventing Stiffness | 82 |

### 6. BALANCE AND STABILITY: PREVENTING FALLS AND INJURIES — 87

| | |
|---|---|
| 6.1 Understanding the Importance of Balance | 88 |
| 6.2 Simple Balance Exercises for Daily Practice | 90 |
| 6.3 Tai Chi for Seniors: Improving Balance and Flexibility | 93 |
| 6.4 Yoga for Balance: Poses and Practices | 96 |
| 6.5 Safety Tips for Balance Exercises | 98 |

### 7. STRENGTH TRAINING: BUILDING MUSCLE SAFELY — 101

| | |
|---|---|
| 7.1 Bodyweight Exercises for Strength | 101 |
| 7.2 Using Resistance Bands: An Affordable Option | 104 |
| 7.3 Light Weight Training: Building Muscle Gradually | 106 |
| 7.4 Blood Flow Restriction Training: A New Approach to Weight Training | 108 |
| 7.5 Strength Training Safety and Modifications | 111 |

### 8. ADVANCED EXERCISE TECHNIQUES: KEEPING IT INTERESTING — 115

| | |
|---|---|
| 8.1 Interactive Element: Personal Aerobics Progress Tracker | 117 |
| 8.2 Elliptical and Treadmill Workouts | 119 |
| 8.3 Vibration Plate: Enhancing Exercise Benefits | 121 |
| 8.4 Aquatic Exercises: Low-Impact, High-Benefit | 123 |
| 8.5 Combining Techniques for a Holistic Routine | 126 |

### 9. HOLISTIC HEALTH: CONNECTING MIND AND BODY — 131

| | |
|---|---|
| 9.1 The Mental Benefits of Regular Exercise | 131 |
| 9.2 Stress Reduction Techniques for Seniors | 134 |

9.3 Mind-Body Exercises: Meditation 136
9.4 The Importance of Sleep and Hydration 137
9.5 Building a Supportive Community 138
9.6 Tracking Progress: Tools and Tips 140
9.7 Inspiring Success Stories 142
9.8 Staying Motivated: Long-Term Health and Wellness 144

Conclusion 147
References 151

## Introduction

I want to tell you a story about Marie. At 68, she felt her age creeping up on her. She struggled with joint pain, low energy, and a few extra pounds that wouldn't budge. She felt trapped in a body that no longer did what she wanted. But then, she decided to make a change. She started with her diet, switching to a Keto plan recommended by a friend who had recently experienced significant weight loss using the diet. Soon after, she began integrating gentle exercises like walking around the block, Tai Chi, and chair yoga. Within months, Marie felt a transformation. Her energy returned, her pain lessened, and she lost that stubborn weight. Today, she feels stronger and more vibrant than she has in years.

Hi, I'm Alex Silver. At 55, I understand firsthand the importance of maintaining a healthy lifestyle as we age. I have dedicated my life to promoting wellness through nutrition and exercise. With a background looking at various diets and personal training that has worked for me, I've spent my time and energy helping seniors regain their health and vitality. My passion stems from my own experiences. I've faced the challenges of aging, and I've seen the power of diet and exercise to turn things around.

This book is for you. It's a guide to help you build strength, balance, flexibility, and a sharp mind. The goal is to empower you to lead a fulfilling, active life. We'll start with diet because getting healthy from the inside out makes everything else easier. Then, we'll explore a variety of exercises tailored to your needs.

Seniors often face unique challenges when it comes to diet and exercise. Metabolic Syndrome affects most seniors in some way. But what exactly is Metabolic Syndrome? According to the NCEP ATP III definition, metabolic syndrome is present if a person meets three or more of the following five criteria:

- Waist circumference over 40 inches (men) or 35 inches (women).
- Blood pressure over 130/85 mmHg.
- Fasting triglyceride (TG) level over 150 mg/dl.
- Fasting high-density lipoprotein (HDL) cholesterol level less than 40 mg/dl (men) or 50 mg/dl (women).
- Fasting blood sugar level over 100 mg/dl (National Cholesterol Education Program [NCEP], 2002).

Please note that LDL cholesterol is not a factor in Metabolic Syndrome.

Metabolic health issues can make weight loss difficult. Chronic pain limits mobility. A lack of motivation can make it challenging to stick to a plan. Did you know that nearly 80% of adults aged 65 and older have at least one chronic condition? And around 60% have at least two (Centers for Disease Control and Prevention [CDC], 2013). These statistics show the urgency of addressing health issues head-on.

In this book, we'll tackle these challenges together. We'll start with unconventional diets like Keto, Carnivore, and Paleo. These diets focus on reducing inflammation and improving metabolic health. Once your body is in a better state, we'll introduce a range of exercises. From walking and aerobics to weight training and aquatic activities, you'll find something that suits your fitness level and interests.

You won't be alone on this journey. We're bringing in insights from respected doctors like Dr. Shawn Baker, Dr. Ken Berry, Dr. Eric Westman, Dr. Annette Bosworth, and Dr. Anthony Chaffee. They'll share their expertise on diet and health, providing valuable advice and tips. For example, Dr. Baker will explain how the Carnivore diet can reduce inflammation (Baker, 2019), while Dr. Berry and Dr. Boz will discuss the benefits of the Keto diet for metabolic health and introduce ideas like intermittent fasting and specific types of fasts (Berry, 2019; Bosworth, 2020).

What makes this book unique is our approach of prioritizing diet first. When you restore your health through nutrition, you'll find it easier to engage in physical activity. This method makes fitness more accessible and effective for seniors. You'll feel the difference when you fuel your body properly, and exercise becomes a joy rather than a chore.

Here's a brief roadmap of what we'll cover:

1. Diet: We'll dive into the principles of Keto, Carnivore, and Paleo diets. You'll learn how to implement these eating plans and the science behind their benefits.
2. Exercise Routines: We'll explore different types of exercises, including walking, aerobics, Tai Chi, yoga, chair exercises, weight training, and more.

3. Balance Training: We'll focus on exercises that improve balance, helping you stay steady and prevent falls.
4. Strength Training: You'll learn about the importance of building muscle and how to do it safely at any age.
5. Advanced Techniques: We'll introduce more advanced exercises like blood flow restriction training and vibration plate use.
6. Holistic Health: We'll touch on the importance of mental well-being, stress management, and sleep.

I encourage you to commit to changing your diet and exercise habits. It's always possible to start living a healthier, more active life. Begin with small steps. Swap out processed foods for whole, nutrient-dense options. Take a short walk each day. Gradually, these small changes will add up to significant improvements.

This journey is about more than just physical health. It's about feeling better, having more energy, and enjoying life to the fullest. When you address your diet first, you create a strong foundation for effective exercise. With expert insights and multiple types of exercises to perform, you'll find a plan that works for you.

So, let's get started. Together, we'll unlock the potential for a healthier, more vibrant you.

# 1

## The Foundation of Health: Understanding Diet and Exercise for Seniors

Think about Jim. At 72, he had resigned himself to his aches, pains, and frequent bouts of fatigue. His doctor had recommended more exercise, but Jim didn't know where to start. Then he met a friend who had recently started a new diet and was seeing incredible benefits. Curious, Jim decided to give it a try. He began with simple dietary changes, cutting out processed foods and sugar and adding more protein and healthy fats. His energy levels soared within weeks, and Jim felt motivated to start walking daily. Soon, Jim was not just walking but also enjoying light strength training, feeling younger and more vibrant than he had in years.

I'm Alex Silver, and like you, I've faced the challenges of aging. At 55, I've made it my mission to help others navigate these years with grace and vitality. With a background in various diets and personal training that works, I've seen firsthand how the proper diet can transform lives, especially when it comes to seniors. This chapter will lay the foundation for your journey toward better health, starting with the crucial role of diet.

## 1.1 Why Diet Comes First: The Foundation of Health

Diet is more than just what you eat; it's the cornerstone of your overall health, especially as you age. When your body is metabolically healthy, everything else falls into place more easily. A metabolically healthy body means your cells function optimally and your energy levels are stable (Feinman et al., 2015). You'll find it easier to engage in physical activities, and your body will recover faster from exercise. Moreover, a good diet reduces inflammation, which is often the root cause of many chronic conditions (Calder, 2020).

The benefits of focusing on diet first are numerous. For starters, a well-structured diet can lead to significant health improvements, making starting an exercise routine much easier. For instance, losing even a small amount of weight can relieve pressure on your joints, making movement less painful (Messier et al., 2013). Better blood sugar regulation means fewer energy crashes, so you'll feel more motivated to stay active (Westman et al., 2018). Improved blood pressure control can reduce the risk of heart disease and stroke (Appel et al., 1997), while removing "brain fog" keeps you sharp and focused.

Let's discuss some practical dietary changes you can make right now. One of the simplest yet most impactful changes is eliminating processed foods. These foods are high in sugars, unhealthy fats, and additives that can wreak havoc on your metabolic health (Monteiro et al., 2018). Instead, focus on increasing your protein intake, such as chicken, fatty red meat, and fish. Proteins are the building blocks of muscle and are crucial for maintaining muscle mass as you age (Phillips, 2017). Healthy fats in foods like fatty meats, fish, avocados, nuts, and olive oil are essential for brain health and hormone production (Yehuda et al., 1999). And, of course, cutting out sugar can have immediate benefits, such as better blood sugar control and reduced inflammation (Lustig et al., 2016).

But how exactly does diet support your exercise efforts? When you fuel your body correctly, you'll have sustained energy during your workouts, making them more effective and enjoyable. Think of it like filling your car with high-quality fuel; it runs smoother and more efficiently. Proper nutrition also means faster recovery times, so you can exercise more frequently without feeling worn out (Kerksick et al., 2017). Improved muscle function is another benefit, as your muscles need the proper nutrients to perform and grow (Phillips, 2017). Lastly, a good diet reduces inflammation and pain, making physical activities less daunting and more attainable (Calder, 2020).

As you embark on this journey, remember that small, consistent changes can lead to significant improvements. Start by making one or two dietary adjustments and gradually build from there. You don't need to overhaul your entire diet overnight. The key is to create sustainable habits supporting your long-term health and well-being. By prioritizing diet, you're laying a solid foundation that will make exercise possible and enjoyable.

## 1.2 Metabolic Health: The Key to Effective Exercise

When we talk about metabolic health, we're referring to how well your body processes and uses energy. This involves several key factors, including blood sugar levels, insulin sensitivity, and cholesterol management. For seniors, maintaining good metabolic health is crucial for engaging in physical activity effectively. Blood sugar levels must be stable to avoid crashes that can sap your energy. Insulin sensitivity, which refers to how responsive your cells are to insulin, is vital for keeping blood sugar levels in check. Poor insulin sensitivity can lead to type 2 diabetes and other metabolic disorders (DeFronzo, 2009). Cholesterol management is equally important, as improper cholesterol levels can increase the risk of heart disease (Grundy, 2016). Please note that we will not obsess about LDL cholesterol; we are more interested in HDL cholesterol and triglycerides.

Poor metabolic health can make exercise a real challenge. If your blood sugar levels are all over the place, you might feel fatigued even before you start your workout. This can lead to a vicious cycle of feeling too tired to exercise, worsening your metabolic issues (Gerstein et al., 2008). Additionally, poor metabolic health can increase your risk of injury. For instance, if your muscles and joints are inflamed, you're more likely to experience pain or even suffer an injury during physical activity (Hotamisligil, 2006). Finally, slower muscle recovery is another issue. When your body isn't metabolically healthy, it takes longer to heal and recover from exercise, making it harder to stick to a regular workout routine (Phillips, 2017).

Diet plays a pivotal role in improving metabolic health. One effective strategy is adopting a low-carb diet, which is shown to help regulate blood sugar levels. According to Dr. Ken Berry, a low-carb diet can improve insulin sensitivity and reduce the risk of type 2 diabetes (Westman et al., 2018). By limiting the intake of carbohydrates, you help your body use fats and proteins more efficiently for energy. Speaking of protein, it's crucial for maintaining muscle mass and supporting metabolic health. Proteins are the building blocks of our muscles, and a higher protein intake can help you feel fuller longer, reducing the urge to snack on unhealthy foods (Phillips, 2017).

Hydration is another crucial element in metabolic health. Drinking enough water helps your body function optimally, aiding digestion and nutrient absorption. Proper hydration can also significantly affect how you feel during exercise. Imagine trying to work out when you're dehydrated; it's like running a car without enough oil. Everything is more challenging, and you're more likely to wear out quickly (Sawka et al., 2007). However, more than hydration is needed. As you change your diet, you will also need to work on keeping your electrolytes in balance, as the dietary changes you are making will cause you to lose vast amounts of water weight in the beginning stages (Phinney & Volek, 2011).

Good metabolic health contributes significantly to overall well-being. When your metabolism is functioning well, you'll notice enhanced mental well-being. Stable blood sugar levels mean fewer mood swings and better mental clarity (Goldstein et al., 2009). You'll also find that you sleep better when your metabolic health is in check. Quality sleep is essential for recovery and overall health (Van Cauter et al., 2008). And let's remember the big picture: increased life expectancy. Studies have shown that good metabolic health can contribute to a longer, healthier life (Ford et al., 2010). Better mental acuity is another benefit, as a healthy metabolism supports brain function, keeping you sharp and focused (Gunstad et al., 2007).

Consider this: improving your metabolic health is like tuning up a car. When everything is running smoothly, the vehicle performs better, has fewer breakdowns, and has a longer lifespan. The same goes for your body. By focusing on metabolic health, you set yourself up for better exercise performance, quicker recovery times, and an overall higher quality of life.

### 1.3 The Role of Nutrition in Aging Well

As we age, our nutritional needs evolve, and meeting these specific requirements becomes crucial for maintaining health and vitality. One of the most important nutrients for seniors is calcium, which plays a vital role in bone health. As we age, our bones lose density, making them more susceptible to fractures and conditions like osteoporosis (Lanham-New et al., 2012). Incorporating calcium-rich foods such as dairy products, fatty meats, and organ meats can help maintain bone strength. Another key nutrient is omega-3 fatty acids, which are essential for heart health. Found in fatty fish like salmon, as well as flaxseeds and walnuts, omega-3s help reduce inflammation, lower blood pressure, and support overall cardiovascular function (Mozaffarian & Wu, 2011).

Adequate protein intake is another cornerstone of senior nutrition. Protein is essential for maintaining muscle mass, which naturally declines with age. This decline can decrease strength and mobility, making daily activities more challenging (Breen & Phillips, 2011). Including protein-rich foods like meats from ruminant animals (beef, lamb, elk, and bison), eggs, fish, and other seafood in your diet can help preserve muscle mass and support overall body maintenance. Antioxidants are also crucial for cellular protection. These compounds, found in colorful fruits and vegetables like berries, citrus fruits, and leafy greens, help combat oxidative stress and inflammation, which can contribute to chronic diseases and aging (Harman, 2003).

Proper nutrition can significantly mitigate many age-related issues. For example, a diet rich in calcium and vitamin D can reduce the risk of osteoporosis by strengthening bones (Lanham-New et al., 2012). Managing arthritis symptoms can be more attainable by incorporating anti-inflammatory foods like turmeric, ginger, and omega-3-rich fish into your meals. These foods can help reduce joint pain and stiffness, making it easier to stay active (Henrotin et al., 2011). Supporting cognitive function is another critical aspect of senior nutrition. Foods high in antioxidants, like blueberries and spinach, can protect brain cells from damage and improve mental sharpness and memory (Joseph et al., 2009).

Creating nutritious meal plans that cater to seniors' needs doesn't have to be complicated. Start by understanding macronutrients—proteins, fats, and carbohydrates—and their role in your diet. Proteins are essential for muscle maintenance, fats provide energy and support cell function, and carbohydrates are the only macronutrient that does not have essential qualities (Eaton et al., 1988). Carbohydrates should be limited and rare in your diet. Aim to incorporate nutrient-dense foods into every meal. This means choosing foods high in vitamins, minerals, and other beneficial compounds relative to their calorie content. For instance, opt for whole grains over refined grains or eliminate grains entirely, and choose fresh fruits and vegetables over processed snacks.

Avoiding empty calories is also crucial. These foods and drinks provide little to no nutritional value, such as sugary beverages, candy, and baked goods (Malik et al., 2010). Instead, focus on whole, unprocessed foods that nourish your body and support your health. Read the labels of foods you choose at the grocery store; if there are more than three ingredients, this isn't real food and contains many empty calories. Practical meal planning tips include preparing meals in advance, using various cooking methods to keep things interesting, and incorporating a mix of protein, healthy fats, and fiber-rich carbohydrates in each meal.

Here are some simple, nutrient-rich recipes to get you started. For breakfast, you might enjoy a hearty omelet filled with bacon, tomatoes, and feta cheese. This dish provides a good mix of protein, healthy fats, and antioxidants. For lunch, consider a baked salmon fillet paired with steamed vegetables like broccoli and carrots. Salmon is an excellent source of omega-3 fatty acids, while vegetables offer fiber and essential vitamins. Dinner could be a delicious steak or lamb chop, rich in protein and iron, served with roasted asparagus and a mixed green salad.

For those following specific dietary plans like Paleo, Keto, or Carnivore, plenty of options align with these principles. On a Paleo diet, you might enjoy grilled chicken with a side of sautéed vegetables seasoned with herbs and olive oil. For a Keto-friendly meal, try a cheese and avocado salad topped with a generous serving of grilled shrimp. Those on a Carnivore diet can keep things simple with a juicy ribeye steak seasoned with salt, pepper, and a butter sauce.

Meeting your nutritional needs through thoughtful meal planning can make a world of difference in how you feel and function each day. Focusing on nutrient-dense foods and balanced meals will help you support your body's unique requirements as you age, helping to maintain strength, vitality, and overall well-being.

### 1.4 Overcoming Common Diet and Exercise Myths

One of the most persistent myths about senior diets is that seniors need less protein. This misconception leads to a host of health issues, from muscle loss to weakened immune function. Research shows that as we age, our bodies actually require more protein to maintain muscle mass and overall health. According to Dr. Ken Berry, a family physician with over two decades of experience, increasing protein intake can help seniors fight off muscle wasting and stay strong (Berry, 2018). It's not just about maintaining muscle mass; protein also plays a vital role in repairing tissues and supporting immune function. So, the next time someone tells you that you don't need much protein, remember that your body begs to differ.

Another common myth is that low-fat diets are best for seniors. This idea stems from outdated nutritional guidelines that link dietary fat to heart disease. However, modern research has debunked this myth. Healthy fats, like those found in red meat, avocados, nuts, and olive oil, are crucial for brain health, hormone production, and even weight management. Cutting out fats can lead to nutrient deficiencies and make you feel unsatisfied, prompting you to overeat. Studies have shown that diets including healthy fats can improve metabolic health and reduce the risk of chronic diseases (Siri-Tarino et al., 2010). So, don't shy away from fats; they are your friends, not foes.

The notion that carbs are necessary is another myth that can be misleading. While carbohydrates are a source of energy, they are not the only source, nor are they always the best source. Low-carb diets improve insulin sensitivity, regulate blood sugar levels, and support weight loss (Westman, 2002). For seniors, managing blood sugar is particularly important to avoid conditions like type 2 diabetes and dementia, which now is sometimes referred to as type 3 diabetes due to the connection between insulin resistance and cognitive decline (de la Monte & Wands, 2008). Carbs are not inherently bad, but the type and amount you consume matter. Focus on carbs like cruciferous vegetables, and consider removing refined carbs and sugars from your diet for better health outcomes.

Regarding exercise, myths abound, particularly the belief that strength training is dangerous for seniors. This myth can be particularly harmful, discouraging an incredibly beneficial activity. Strength training helps maintain muscle mass, improves bone density, and boosts metabolism. According to various studies, older adults who engage in strength training experience fewer falls, better mobility, and improved overall health (Nelson et al., 2004). The key is to start with light weights and gradually increase intensity under proper guidance. Proper technique and safety precautions make strength training safe and highly effective for seniors.

Another damaging myth is that it's too late to start exercising. This belief can rob you of the incredible benefits of being active. No matter your age, exercise can improve your quality of life. It's never too late to start moving. Whether it's a gentle walk around the block, a yoga class, or some light weightlifting, every bit of movement helps. Incremental progress is the name of the game here. Start small and gradually increase your activity level. Even modest amounts of exercise can lead to significant health improvements, including better cardiovascular health, increased strength, and enhanced mental well-being (Warburton et al., 2006).

The idea that cardio is the only important exercise is another myth that needs busting. While cardiovascular exercise is vital for heart health, it's not the only type of exercise that matters. A balanced exercise routine includes strength training, flexibility exercises, and balance training. Each type of exercise offers unique benefits. For example, strength training builds muscle, flexibility exercises improve range of motion, and balance exercises help prevent falls. A well-rounded exercise program will address all these areas, providing comprehensive health benefits (ACSM, 2011).

Scientific research supports these points. Studies on protein needs for seniors have shown that higher protein intake leads to better muscle maintenance and overall health (Breen & Phillips, 2011). Research on the benefits of strength training for older adults highlights improved bone density and reduced risk of falls (Nelson et al., 2004). Additionally, balanced exercise routines that include various types of activities offer the most comprehensive health benefits. It's about creating a routine that addresses all aspects of health, from cardiovascular fitness to muscle strength and flexibility.

Changing your mindset is also crucial. It's easy to get stuck in the belief that change is hard or that it's too late. However, seniors worldwide are proving there is always time to adopt healthier habits.

Take the story of Jack, who, at 75, decided to start a fitness routine after a lifetime of inactivity. He began with a simple walk around the block several times a week. He then started chair exercises and gradually moved on to more challenging activities. Today, Jack is more active and healthier than he was in his 50s. His story is a testament to the power of incremental progress and its positive impacts on daily living. Small steps lead to significant changes, and it's never too late to start.

## 1.5 Setting Realistic and Achievable Health Goals

Imagine you're setting out on a road trip. You wouldn't just hop into the car and start driving aimlessly, would you? You'd want a clear destination, a map, and checkpoints along the way to ensure you're heading in the right direction. The same principle applies to your health goals. Setting realistic and achievable health goals is like plotting your course on a map. It gives you clear direction, helps you measure progress, and keeps you motivated.

When you have a specific goal in mind, it's easier to focus your efforts. Instead of vaguely aiming to "get healthier," you might set a goal to walk 20 minutes daily. This clear direction helps you know exactly what you must do daily to move closer to your goal. It also makes it easier to track your progress. It feels good when you can see that you've walked 20 minutes every day for a week. That sense of accomplishment can boost your motivation and encourage you to keep going (Locke & Latham, 2002).

To set practical goals, use the SMART method: Specific, Measurable, Achievable, Relevant, and Time-bound. Start by defining your exact health objectives. Instead of saying, "I want to lose weight," specify, "I intend to lose 10 pounds." Next, make your goal measurable. Use tangible metrics like pounds lost, minutes walked, or blood pressure readings to track your progress and see how far you've come. Your goals should also be achievable. If you've been sedentary for a while, aiming to run a marathon in a month isn't realistic. Instead, aim to walk 15 minutes daily and gradually increase your activity level.

Relevance is another important factor. Your goals should be meaningful and align with your overall health aspirations. If reducing your blood pressure is important to you, set a goal to lower it by 10 points (American Heart Association [AHA], 2017). Finally, make your goals time-bound. Setting a deadline adds a sense of urgency and helps you stay focused. For example, aim to lose 5% of your body weight in three months. This gives you a clear timeframe to work within and helps you stay on track.

Let's look at some practical examples of short-term and long-term goals. A short-term goal might be to walk for 20 minutes daily for the next two weeks, which is specific, measurable, achievable, relevant, and time-bound. An intermediate goal could be losing 5% of your body weight over the next three months, giving you a clear target and enough time to make steady progress. A long-term goal might be to reduce your blood pressure by 10 points within six months. This specific and measurable goal gives you a reasonable timeframe to achieve it (National Institutes of Health [NIH], 2016).

Flexibility is crucial in goal-setting. Life happens, and sometimes you need to adjust your goals. Regular self-assessment helps you stay on track and make necessary changes. For instance, if walking 20 minutes a day is too challenging, start with 10 minutes and gradually increase. Celebrate small victories along the way. Every step forward, no matter how small, is progress. If you lose a pound or manage to walk every day for a week, give yourself credit.

These small wins build momentum and keep you motivated (Bandura, 1997).

Reevaluating your objectives is also important. As you make progress, you might find that your initial goals need adjustment. If you've reached your short-term goal of walking 20 minutes a day, set a new goal to walk 30 minutes. If you've successfully lowered your blood pressure by 10 points, aim for another 5-point reduction. Adjusting your goals keeps you moving forward and ensures you're constantly challenging yourself.

Setting realistic and achievable health goals is a powerful tool for maintaining motivation and achieving success. It provides clear direction, allows you to measure your progress, and enhances your motivation. Using the SMART method, setting practical goals, and being flexible can create a roadmap to better health. Remember to celebrate your achievements, no matter how small, and keep reassessing your goals to ensure they remain relevant and attainable.

As you progress, consider your goals as stepping stones toward better health. Each goal you achieve is a step closer to a more active, vibrant life. Embrace the process, stay flexible, and keep celebrating your progress. Your health is a journey; with each step, you're building a stronger, healthier future.

# 2

# Unconventional Diets: Exploring Keto, Carnivore, and Paleo

Imagine Jim, a 65-year-old retiree who struggled with weight gain and low energy. He was skeptical about diets until he stumbled upon the Keto diet. Jim decided to try it, and within a few weeks, he noticed significant changes. His energy levels soared, he shed some pounds, and he felt more mentally alert. Stories like Jim's illustrate the transformative power of the Keto diet, particularly for seniors seeking to regain control over their health.

## 2.1 The Keto Diet: High Fat, Low Carb for Seniors

The Keto diet revolves around a simple yet powerful principle: consuming high fat, moderate protein, and low carbohydrates. By drastically reducing your carb intake, your body enters a state called ketosis. In ketosis, your body becomes incredibly efficient at burning fat for energy instead of relying on glucose from carbs (Paoli, Rubini, Volek, & Grimaldi, 2013). This metabolic state helps in weight loss and offers numerous health benefits.

One of the standout benefits of the Keto diet for seniors is improved cognitive function. Our brains can become more susceptible to memory issues and cognitive decline as we age. Studies have shown that ketones, the engine of fat metabolism, provide an efficient and stable energy source for the brain, enhancing mental clarity and memory (Cunnane et al., 2016). This is particularly important for seniors at risk of conditions like Alzheimer's disease, as a low-carb diet has been shown to improve memory function in older adults with mild cognitive impairment (Taylor et al., 2018).

Another significant advantage of the Keto diet is enhanced energy levels. Unlike the energy rollercoaster you experience with high-carb diets, ketosis provides a steady and sustained energy supply, which is a game-changer for seniors who often struggle with fatigue. Imagine going through your day with consistent energy, allowing you to engage in physical activities and hobbies without feeling drained (Westman, Mavropoulos, Yancy, & Volek, 2003).

Better blood sugar control is a critical benefit of the Keto diet. Many seniors have type 2 diabetes or prediabetes, and managing blood sugar levels is paramount. By reducing carbohydrate intake, the Keto diet helps stabilize blood sugar levels and improve insulin sensitivity (Boden, Sargrad, Homko, Mozzoli, & Stein, 2005). This can lead to fewer blood sugar spikes and crashes, making it easier to manage diabetes and reduce medication dependence.

Weight management is another area in which the Keto diet shines. Many seniors find it challenging to lose weight due to slower metabolism and decreased physical activity. The Keto diet promotes fat loss by shifting your body into a fat-burning mode, which leads to significant weight loss, particularly around the midsection, which is often the most stubborn area for many people (Bueno, de Melo, de Oliveira, & da Rocha Ataide, 2013).

Additionally, the diet's high-fat content helps keep you feeling full and satisfied, reducing the urge to snack on unhealthy foods.

So, what can you eat on a Keto diet? The focus is on nutrient-dense, low-carb foods that support overall health. Avocados are a Keto superstar, packed with healthy fats, fiber, and essential vitamins. Nuts and seeds are excellent for snacking and add a satisfying crunch to meals. Olive oil is a fantastic source of healthy fats, perfect for dressing salads or cooking. Fatty fish like salmon and mackerel provide omega-3 fatty acids crucial for heart health. Meats like beef and lamb are also stars as long as you choose the fattier cuts of those foods. Low-carb vegetables, such as spinach, kale, and broccoli, offer essential nutrients without the carb load.

To help you get started, here's a sample Keto meal plan for a week:

- Breakfast: Scrambled eggs with spinach and avocado. This meal is rich in protein and healthy fats, giving you a solid start to your day.
- Lunch: Grilled chicken salad with olive oil dressing. This dish combines lean protein, healthy fats, and plenty of greens, keeping you full and energized through the afternoon.
- Dinner: Baked salmon with asparagus. This meal provides a hefty amount of omega-3 fatty acids and fiber, promoting heart health and digestion.
- Snacks: Cheese sticks, almonds, or pecans. These options are easy to carry and provide a satisfying mix of fats and protein, perfect for curbing hunger between meals.

Starting a new diet can be daunting, but the benefits of the Keto diet make it worth considering. Focusing on high-fat, low-carb foods can improve your cognitive function, boost energy levels, better manage your blood sugar, and achieve weight loss goals. It's a powerful tool for seniors looking to enhance their health and enjoy a more active, fulfilling life.

If you find it helpful, consider using a food journal to track your meals and progress, so you stay accountable and make adjustments as needed. Remember, the journey to better health is a marathon, not a sprint. Small, consistent changes can lead to significant improvements over time.

## 2.2 Carnivore Diet: Meat-Centric Nutrition

Imagine switching to a diet where you primarily eat meat. That's the essence of the Carnivore diet. It's a straightforward approach that eliminates plant-based foods entirely, focusing solely on animal products. The idea is to consume foods that our ancestors might have eaten, relying on meats like beef, bison, pork, fish, and eggs. It's a radical shift from the conventional wisdom that promotes a balanced diet with fruits and vegetables. But the simplicity of the Carnivore diet can be incredibly appealing, especially for those who find meal planning overwhelming.

One of the remarkable benefits of the Carnivore diet is its potential to reduce inflammation. Chronic inflammation is common among seniors, contributing to conditions like arthritis and cardiovascular disease. By eliminating plant foods that may cause inflammation, such as grains, sugar, and certain vegetables, the Carnivore diet can help alleviate these symptoms (Mikovits & Heckenlively, 2020). Dr. Shawn Baker, a prominent advocate of this diet, has reported numerous cases where individuals experienced significant reductions in joint pain and swelling, making a world of difference in their daily comfort and mobility (Baker, 2019).

Another advantage is the simplicity of meal planning. With the Carnivore diet, you don't have to worry about counting calories or balancing macronutrients because it is tough for most people to overeat protein (Naiman, 2019). You focus on consuming high-quality meats and animal products, which can make meal preparation straightforward and stress-free. This can be particularly beneficial for seniors who may not have the energy or desire to spend much time in the kitchen. The diet's simplicity can also make it easier to stick to, reducing the likelihood of falling off the wagon.

Mental sharpness is another benefit that many people on the Carnivore diet report. Our brains thrive on healthy fats and proteins, and the Carnivore diet provides these in abundance. The steady supply of nutrients can enhance cognitive function, helping you stay sharp, which is particularly important as we age, as maintaining mental acuity can significantly impact our quality of life (Smith & Hiltz, 2018). Many followers of the Carnivore diet, including seniors, have reported feeling more alert and mentally clear, which can improve overall well-being.

Weight reduction is often a primary goal for those adopting the Carnivore diet. Cutting out carbohydrates shifts your body into a fat-burning mode, similar to the Keto diet, and this can lead to significant weight loss, especially in visceral fat, often the most challenging fat for seniors to lose (Volek & Phinney, 2011). The diet's high-protein content helps keep you full and satisfied, reducing the urge to snack. It is also very challenging to overeat meat, and this fact can make weight loss more manageable and sustainable over the long term.

So, what can you eat on the Carnivore diet? The focus is on nutrient-dense, high-quality animal products. You can eat it if it walks, runs, flies, swims, crawls, or slithers. You can also enjoy any byproducts, such as dairy, from these animals. Beef is a staple, providing essential nutrients like iron, zinc, and omega-3 fatty acids. Organ meats like liver and kidneys are incredibly nutrient-dense, offering vitamins and minerals that are challenging to find in other foods (Norris, 2020). Include cheese and other dairy products, also as they provide calcium and healthy fats. Eggs are another excellent choice, packed with protein and essential nutrients. Fish and seafood offer a great source of omega-3 fatty acids, which are crucial for health.

Like any diet, the Carnivore approach comes with its challenges. Initial digestive issues are common as your body adapts to the new way of eating, including bloating, constipation, or diarrhea. To mitigate these issues, start slowly and give your body time to adjust (Baker, 2019). Electrolyte imbalance is another genuine concern. The Carnivore diet can lead to a drop in electrolytes like sodium, potassium, and magnesium as your body eliminates vast amounts of stored water as you begin this diet (Naiman, 2019). Make sure to consume enough salt and consider supplements if needed. Social dining scenarios can be tricky, as the Carnivore diet is quite restrictive. Plan ahead by checking restaurant menus or bringing your own food to gatherings.

To help you get started, here's a sample Carnivore meal plan for a week:

- Breakfast: Enjoy bacon and eggs. This meal is rich in protein and healthy fats, providing a satisfying start to your day.
- Lunch: Try hamburger patties (no bun) with cheese. This combination offers a good mix of nutrients and keeps you full.
- Dinner: Savor a ribeye steak with butter. This meal is not only delicious but also packed with essential nutrients.

- Eliminate snacks to maintain the integrity of the diet and allow your body to fully adapt to this new way of eating.

Switching to the Carnivore diet can be a significant change, but the potential benefits make it worth considering. By focusing on high-quality animal products, you can reduce inflammation, simplify meal planning, improve mental outlook, and achieve your weight loss goals. With some planning and patience, you can successfully navigate the challenges and reap the rewards of this meat-centric approach.

## 2.3 Paleo Diet: Eating Like Our Ancestors

Think back to a time before processed foods, when our ancestors thrived on what they could hunt and gather. This is the essence of the Paleo diet. It's about returning to a way of eating that focuses on whole, unprocessed foods. The Paleo diet eliminates grains, legumes, and processed sugars, aiming to mimic the diet of our Paleolithic ancestors. The idea is that our bodies are better adapted to this type of diet, leading to improved health and well-being (Cordain, 2011).

The Paleo diet offers several benefits for seniors. One of the most notable is better digestion. Many older adults struggle with digestive issues, often caused by processed foods and grains. By focusing on whole foods, you can reduce inflammation in the gut and improve overall digestive health. Fresh fruits and vegetables are fiber-rich, aiding digestion and promoting regular bowel movements (Wolf, 2010). Lean meats provide essential proteins without the additives found in processed meats.

Another significant advantage is enhanced immune function. The Paleo diet is rich in vitamins, minerals, and antioxidants that support a robust immune system. Fresh fruits and vegetables, such as berries, leafy greens, and citrus fruits, are packed with nutrients that help fight off infections and keep your immune system strong. Lean meats like chicken and turkey offer high-quality protein without the unhealthy fats found in processed meats. Nuts and seeds provide essential fatty acids that support cellular health and function (Sisson, 2011).

Stable energy levels are a crucial benefit of the Paleo diet. Unlike diets high in refined carbs and sugars, which can cause energy spikes and crashes, the Paleo diet provides a steady supply of energy throughout the day. Healthy fats from sources like olive oil, coconut oil, and avocados help keep you full and satisfied, preventing the mid-afternoon energy slump that often leads to unhealthy snacking (Cordain & Friel, 2005). This consistency can be particularly beneficial for seniors who need consistent energy levels to stay active and engaged in daily activities.

Think fresh and natural when it comes to foods allowed on the Paleo diet. Fresh fruits and vegetables are a cornerstone, offering essential vitamins, minerals, and fiber. Meats like chicken, turkey, and grass-fed beef provide high-quality protein without the unhealthy fats found in processed meats. Nuts and seeds are excellent for snacking and adding a satisfying crunch to meals. Healthy fats, like those found in olive, coconut, and palm oils, are crucial for brain health and hormone production (Wolf, 2010). These foods nourish your body and support overall health and well-being.

To help you get started, here's a sample Paleo meal plan for a week. Try a smoothie with berries, spinach, and almond milk for breakfast. This nutrient-packed drink offers balanced protein, healthy fats, and fiber to start your day on the right foot. For lunch, turkey lettuce wraps with avocado make a delicious and satisfying meal. The lean protein from the turkey and the healthy fats from the avocado will keep you full and energized. Dinner could be grilled chicken with roasted vegetables. This meal provides a hefty dose of protein and fiber, promoting muscle maintenance and digestive health. For snacks, consider coconut flakes and carrot sticks. These options are easy to prepare and offer a satisfying crunch without the added sugars and unhealthy fats found in processed snacks.

Adopting the Paleo diet can be a significant shift, but its potential benefits are worth considering. Focusing on whole, unprocessed foods can improve digestion, enhance immune function, and maintain stable energy levels. This diet supports overall health and helps you feel more vibrant and engaged in your daily life. With a bit of planning and commitment, you can successfully navigate the transition to a Paleo lifestyle and enjoy its many benefits.

Stay organized by using a meal-planning checklist and ensure you have all the ingredients you need for your Paleo meals. Remember, the key to success is consistency. Small, daily changes can lead to significant improvements in your health and well-being over time. So, take it one meal at a time and enjoy the journey back to a more natural way of eating.

## 2.4 Comparing the Diets: Which One is Right for You?

Each diet—Keto, Carnivore, and Paleo—has its own principles, main food groups, and health benefits, making them unique yet effective in their own ways. The Keto diet hinges on high fat, moderate protein, and low-carb intake. This approach forces the body into ketosis, burning fat for energy instead of carbohydrates. The main food groups here include avocados, nuts, seeds, olive oil, fatty fish, meat, and low-carb vegetables. The health benefits are impressive: improved cognitive function, enhanced energy levels, better blood sugar control, and effective weight management (Westman, Phinney, & Volek, 2007).

The Carnivore diet, on the other hand, is all about simplicity. It eliminates plant-based foods entirely, focusing on animal products like grass-fed beef, organ meats, cheese, eggs, and fish. This diet can significantly reduce inflammation, simplify meal planning, improve mental clarity, and aid in weight reduction (Baker, 2019). It's straightforward: you eat meat and animal products, and that's it.

The Paleo diet takes a more balanced approach by mimicking the eating habits of our ancestors. It emphasizes whole foods and avoids processed foods and grains. Core foods include fresh fruits and vegetables, lean meats, nuts, seeds, and healthy fats like olive oil and coconut oil. The health benefits are wide-ranging, including better digestion, enhanced immune function, and stable energy levels (Cordain, 2010).

When choosing a diet, consider your personal health goals. Are you looking to lose weight, improve mental clarity, or manage a chronic condition like diabetes? Each diet offers different benefits that can align with these goals. Dietary preferences are also crucial. Do you enjoy a variety of foods, or do you prefer simplicity? Existing health conditions can play a significant role, too. For example, the Carnivore diet might be beneficial if you have inflammatory issues (Baker, 2019). Keto could be the way to go if you need better blood sugar control (Westman et al., 2007).

Let's weigh the pros and cons of each diet. The Keto diet is highly effective for weight loss and offers numerous health benefits, but it can be restrictive. You have to limit your carb intake significantly, which means giving up many foods you might love (Westman et al., 2007). The Carnivore diet is simple and straightforward, making meal planning a breeze. However, it lacks variety and can be challenging to stick to long-term (Baker, 2019). The Paleo diet is balanced and nutrient-dense, offering a wide range of foods. But it can be time-consuming to prepare meals from scratch, primarily if you're used to convenience foods (Cordain, 2010).

Real-life success stories can be incredibly motivating. Take Sarah, for instance, who followed the Keto diet. She lost 30 pounds and reported improved mental clarity and energy levels. Her blood sugar levels stabilized, and she felt more in control of her health. Then there's Mark, who embraced the simplicity of the Carnivore diet. He saw a dramatic reduction in his chronic joint pain and found the diet easy to stick to because it eliminated the need for complex meal prep. Lastly, consider Linda, who opted for the Paleo diet. She experienced better digestion, enhanced immune function, and stable energy levels. Linda loved the variety of foods she could eat and found the diet sustainable for the long term.

Each of these stories highlights different aspects of how these diets can transform your life. Improved mobility is a common theme, as reducing inflammation and losing weight can make moving around easier (Cordain, 2010; Westman et al., 2007). Enhanced mental clarity is another benefit, particularly with Keto and Carnivore diets, which provide the brain with a steady supply of ketones for fuel (Baker, 2019; Westman et al., 2007). All three diets often show weight loss achievements, as they help shift the body into fat-burning mode. Improved metabolic health is a significant outcome, especially important for seniors managing chronic conditions like diabetes, hypertension, and obesity.

Considering these points, think about what best aligns with your lifestyle and health goals. Each diet has strengths and potential drawbacks, so choose one you feel confident you can stick to. Whether it's the high-fat, low-carb approach of Keto, the simplicity of Carnivore, or the balanced, whole-food focus of

Paleo, you have options that can cater to your needs and preferences. Your health journey is unique, and finding the proper diet can set the stage for a more vibrant, active life.

## 2.5 Transitioning to a New Diet: Tips and Tricks

Switching to a new diet can feel overwhelming, but taking it step-by-step can make the process smoother and more sustainable. Start with gradual dietary changes to ease your body into the new eating habits. For instance, if you're moving to the Keto diet, slowly reduce your carbohydrate intake while increasing healthy fats to allow your body time to adjust, making the transition less jarring (Westman, Phinney, & Volek, 2007). Keeping a food journal can be incredibly helpful during this phase. Write down what you eat, how it makes you feel, and any changes in your energy levels or mood to keep you accountable and help you identify foods that work best for you (Berry, 2019).

Seeking support from a nutritionist can make a world of difference. A professional can provide personalized advice tailored to your specific needs and health conditions. They can help you navigate the intricacies of your new diet, offer meal-planning tips, and ensure you're meeting all your nutritional requirements (Bosworth, 2020). Having an expert in your corner can boost your confidence and make the transition less daunting. Locating a nutritionist that supports your chosen diet can take time, so make sure you choose your nutritionist wisely.

You might encounter some common obstacles as you adapt to your new diet. Cravings can be challenging, especially for foods you're trying to eliminate. To manage them, ensure you have healthy, satisfying alternatives readily available. For instance, grab a handful of berries or a small piece of dark chocolate if you're craving something sweet (Berry, 2019). Staying hydrated also helps, as thirst can sometimes be mistaken for hunger (Westman et al., 2007). Restaurants can be challenging as many of their menu items are high in carbohydrates. Don't hesitate to ask for modifications to fit your dietary needs.

Monitoring your progress is crucial for staying on track and making necessary adjustments. Regular check-ins can help you assess how well your new diet works for you. Pay attention to how you feel physically and mentally. Are you experiencing more energy? Is your mood improving? Adjusting your macronutrient ratios based on these observations can optimize your diet for better results (Chaffee, 2021). You should tweak your fat and protein intake if you're not losing weight as expected.

Staying motivated and committed to your new diet can be one of the most significant challenges but also the most rewarding. Setting short-term goals can provide a sense of achievement and keep you focused (Berry, 2019). For example, stick to your new diet for two weeks without cheating. Celebrate milestones, no matter how small they may seem. Did you resist a craving or stick to your meal plan for a week? That's worth celebrating! Finding a community for support can also be incredibly motivating. Whether it's online forums, local groups, or diet-specific social media communities, connecting with others on the same path can offer encouragement and advice (Bosworth, 2020).

As you transition to your new diet, remember that it's a process, not a race. Small, consistent changes can significantly improve your health and well-being. By taking gradual steps, keeping a food journal, seeking professional support, and staying focused on your goals, you can successfully navigate the challenges and reap the benefits of your new way of eating. Your journey to better health is unique, and finding the proper diet can set the stage for a more vibrant, active life.

The next chapter will explore professional advice from prominent social media doctors who embrace these diets. We will explore each doctor's perspective on low-carb diets and how following them can enhance your health. We will take a quick look at each of these professionals' journeys with these diets and how they have been able to change the lives of their patients and their own health. We will not provide any specific medical advice as we explore how these doctors are making a difference in people's lives, only their experiences as they have worked with patients and seen remarkable results.

# 3

# Doctor-Approved Diets: Insights from the Experts

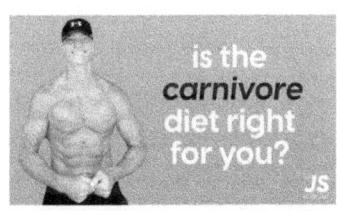

## 3.1 Dr. Shawn Baker - Coined the Phrase "Carnivore Diet"

Imagine you're sitting down with Dr. Shawn Baker, a well-known orthopedic surgeon who has dedicated his last 10 years to transforming lives through nutrition. Dr. Baker isn't your typical doctor; he's a former orthopedic surgeon, a competitive athlete, and a staunch advocate for the Carnivore diet. His journey into this unconventional diet began with his own health struggles. Like many of his patients, he faced joint pain and inflammation, which hindered his athletic performance. Motivated to find a solution, he delved into nutrition science and discovered the potential benefits of an all-meat diet. His personal success with the Carnivore diet led him to research its effects more deeply and share his findings with the world in his best-selling book *The Carnivore Diet* (Baker, 2019).

Dr. Baker's qualifications are impressive. He has over two decades of experience in the medical field. His professional background gives him a unique perspective on the impact of diet on musculoskeletal health. Over the years, Dr. Baker has become a leading voice in the Carnivore community, authoring the book *The Carnivore Diet* and co-founding the website MeatRx.com, a platform dedicated to providing resources and support for those interested in this dietary approach (MeatRx, n.d.). His research contributions and numerous publications have helped shed light on the science behind the Carnivore diet, making it more accessible to the public. Let's not forget his latest endeavor in the medical world, Revero Health, which seeks to provide personalized care for metabolic and autoimmune conditions (Revero Health, n.d.).

According to Dr. Baker, the fundamental principles of the Carnivore diet are straightforward yet powerful. The diet focuses exclusively on nutrient-dense animal products, eliminating all plant-based foods, which means your meals will consist of meats like beef, lamb, pork, and fish, along with other animal products such as eggs and cheese. The idea is to provide your body with all the essential nutrients it needs while minimizing potential irritants and inflammatory substances found in plant foods (Baker, 2019). Doing so can reduce inflammation, improve muscle mass, and enhance mental clarity.

One of Dr. Baker's most significant benefits of the Carnivore diet is its ability to reduce inflammation. Chronic inflammation is a common problem, especially as we age. It's linked to a host of health issues, including arthritis, cardiovascular disease, and even cognitive decline (Baker, 2019). When we eliminate plant foods that can trigger inflammation, the Carnivore diet helps to soothe the body's inflammatory responses. Dr. Baker has seen countless patients experience relief from joint pain and other inflammatory conditions after adopting this way of eating.

Enhancing muscle mass and strength is another critical benefit. Maintaining muscle mass becomes increasingly important for overall health and mobility as we age. The Carnivore diet is rich in high-quality proteins and essential amino acids vital for muscle growth and repair. Dr. Baker himself, an accomplished athlete, has experienced firsthand how this diet can support athletic performance and muscle maintenance. This means better strength, improved mobility, and reduced risk of falls and fractures for seniors (Baker, 2019).

Mental clarity is a benefit that many people might not immediately associate with diet, but Dr. Baker emphasizes its importance. Our brains need a steady supply of nutrients to function optimally, and the Carnivore diet provides these in abundance. Many followers of the diet report enhanced focus, better memory, and overall improved cognitive function (Baker, 2019). Removing "brain fog" can be particularly beneficial for seniors, as maintaining mental acuity is crucial for independence and quality of life.

One of the more practical aspects of the Carnivore diet is its simplicity in meal planning. Without the need to balance various food groups, meal preparation becomes straightforward and stress-free. This can be a significant advantage for those who find traditional meal planning overwhelming. Dr. Baker points out that the diet's simplicity makes it easier to stick to, reducing the likelihood of falling off track (Baker, 2019).

Dr. Baker offers several practical tips for those considering the Carnivore diet to ease the transition. First, start slowly and gradually increase your meat intake, which allows your body to adapt without overwhelming your digestive system. It's also important to ensure variety in your meat sources. Incorporating different types of meat, such as beef, lamb, and fish, ensures you receive a broad spectrum of nutrients. Staying hydrated and monitoring electrolyte levels is crucial, as the diet can change fluid and mineral balance. If necessary, drinking plenty of water and considering supplements can help maintain proper hydration and electrolyte balance (Baker, 2019).

Social dining can be challenging for the Carnivore diet, but Dr. Baker has some advice. Plan ahead by checking restaurant menus online and choosing places that offer carnivore-friendly options. Feel free to ask for modifications to fit your dietary needs. While it might initially feel awkward, your health is worth the effort (Baker, 2019).

To help you navigate these challenges, consider creating a checklist for your transition to the Carnivore diet:

Carnivore Diet Transition Checklist:

- Gradually increase meat intake
- Ensure variety in meat sources
- Stay hydrated and monitor electrolytes
- Plan social dining situations
- Keep a food journal to track progress

Dr. Baker's insights provide a comprehensive guide to adopting the Carnivore diet. Focusing on nutrient-dense animal products can reduce inflammation, enhance muscle mass, improve mental clarity, and simplify meal planning. His practical advice makes navigating the challenges and reaping the benefits of this unique dietary approach easier.

## 3.2 Dr. Ken Berry on the Keto/Carnivore Diet

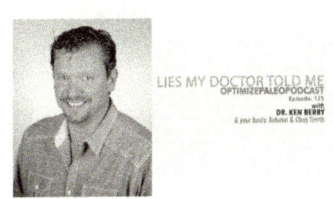

You might have come across Dr. Ken Berry if you've ever looked into low-carb diets. He has a background in family medicine and over two decades of experience treating patients in Tennessee (Berry, 2017). His journey to adopting, at first, a low-carb diet, then a keto/ketovore diet, both personally and professionally, is marked by curiosity and a drive to improve patient outcomes. Dr. Berry struggled with his own weight and health issues for years before discovering the benefits of a low-carb, high-fat diet. His health transformation ignited his passion to share his findings with others (Berry, 2017). He's an accomplished author, and his best-seller is *Lies My Doctor Told Me* (Berry, 2017). He has produced countless YouTube videos and contributed significantly to the low-carb community, where his practical advice and no-nonsense approach have helped many people improve their health.

Regarding the Keto/Ketovore diet, Dr. Berry emphasizes a few core principles. The diet consists of consuming high fat, moderate protein, and very low carbohydrates. This macronutrient composition shifts your body into a state called ketosis (Berry, 2017). In ketosis, your body becomes incredibly efficient at burning fat for energy instead of relying on glucose from carbs. This metabolic state not only aids in weight loss but also provides a steady energy supply, minimizing the peaks and troughs often experienced with high-carb diets (Volek & Phinney, 2012). Another fundamental aspect of the Keto diet, as promoted by Dr. Berry, is the focus on whole, unprocessed foods. He stresses the importance of eliminating sugars, grains, and processed foods from your diet, replacing them with nutrient-dense options like avocados, nuts, seeds, and fatty fish (Berry, 2017).

Dr. Berry has observed numerous health improvements in his patients and himself on the Keto/Ketovore diet. One of the most noticeable benefits is weight loss and fat reduction. Many seniors struggle with weight management, but the Keto diet can make a significant difference (Saslow et al., 2018). By reducing carbohydrate intake and increasing healthy fats, your body shifts into fat-burning mode, leading to steady and sustainable weight loss (Volek & Phinney, 2012). Better blood sugar control is another crucial benefit. For those dealing with type 2 diabetes or prediabetes, managing blood sugar levels is a constant challenge. The Keto diet helps stabilize blood sugar and improve insulin sensitivity, making it easier to manage diabetes and reduce medication dependence (Saslow et al., 2018).

Increased energy levels are also an expected outcome. Unlike the energy rollercoaster of high-carb diets, ketosis provides a steady, reliable energy source, which is a game-changer for seniors who often feel fatigued (Volek & Phinney, 2012). Imagine going through your day with consistent energy, allowing you to engage in physical activities, hobbies, and social interactions without feeling drained. Improved mental health is another significant benefit. The brain thrives on ketones, the byproducts of fat metabolism, which can enhance cognitive function and mental clarity (Newport et al., 2015). Many people on the Keto diet report feeling more focused and alert, which can be particularly beneficial for maintaining mental acuity as you age (Newport et al., 2015).

Dr. Berry offers several practical tips to help you succeed on the Keto/Ketovore diet. One key piece of advice is to eat until you are "comfortably stuffed." Following this advice by eating whole, mostly animal-based foods, you will find that you don't need to eat constantly. Tracking your macronutrient ratios can also be incredibly helpful as that keeps you accountable and helps you make adjustments as needed (Berry, 2017).

Incorporating fats into your diet is crucial for success in keto/ketovore. Foods like fatty red meat, seafood like salmon and mackerel, avocados, olive oil, and nuts, including almonds and pecans, are excellent sources of healthy fats that can keep you feeling full and satisfied (Volek & Phinney, 2012). These fats provide a steady energy source and support overall health. Addressing the "Keto flu" is another important aspect. When you first start the Keto/Ketovore diet, you might experience symptoms like headaches, fatigue, and irritability as your body adjusts to burning fat for fuel (Saslow et al., 2018). Dr. Berry recommends staying well-hydrated, increasing your salt intake, and getting enough electrolytes to mitigate these symptoms (Berry, 2017).

Keto/Ketovore Diet Food Diary Template: • Breakfast: Record your meal and macronutrient breakdown.

• Lunch: Note what you ate and how it made you feel.

• Dinner: Track your evening meal and any snacks.

• Hydration: Keep a log of your water and electrolyte intake.

• Overall Feelings: Reflect on your energy levels, mood, and any symptoms.

Dr. Berry's insights and practical advice make the Keto/Ketovore diet accessible and achievable. By focusing on high fat and protein coupled with a low carb intake, you can experience significant health improvements (Berry, 2017).

## 3.3 Dr. Eric Westman's Approach to Low-Carb Living

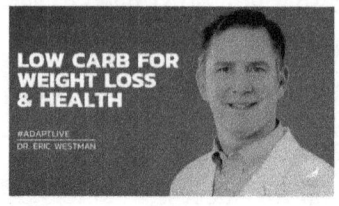

Dr. Eric Westman has made significant strides in the field of low-carb diets. With over 25 years of experience in low-carb research and practice, Dr. Westman is a renowned expert who has dedicated his career to understanding and promoting the benefits of low-carb living. He is an internist and researcher at Duke University, where he has conducted extensive clinical studies on the effects of low-carb diets on metabolic conditions (Westman et al., 2008). His work is widely respected in medical circles, and he has collaborated with low-carbohydrate pioneers like Dr. Atkins (Westman, 2017). Dr. Westman's contributions to developing low-carb dietary guidelines have helped countless individuals improve their health and quality of life. He is also an accomplished author with some titles worth exploring, *End Your Carb Confusion* and *Keto Clarity* (Westman, 2020; Westman & Moore, 2014).

Dr. Westman's low-carb guidelines are both practical and effective. He recommends limiting carbohydrate intake to specific grams per day, typically around 20-50 grams, depending on individual health goals and metabolic conditions. This restriction helps shift the body from burning glucose for energy to burning fat (Volek & Phinney, 2012). Dr. Westman emphasizes the importance of whole foods and balanced nutrition. Instead of relying on processed low-carb products, he advocates for natural, nutrient-dense foods that provide essential vitamins and minerals (Westman, 2020). Protein and healthy fats are crucial components of his dietary recommendations. Foods like red meats, fish, eggs, nuts, and avocados are staples in this approach, ensuring you get the necessary nutrients to support overall health (Westman, 2017).

Clinical findings from Dr. Westman's practice provide compelling evidence of the benefits of a low-carb lifestyle. One notable case study involves a patient who struggled with obesity and type 2 diabetes. After adopting Dr. Westman's low-carb guidelines, the patient experienced significant weight loss and improved blood sugar control (Westman et al., 2008). Within months, they were able to reduce their reliance on medication and felt more energetic. Another patient testimonial highlights improvements in metabolic health markers. This individual saw a reduction in cholesterol levels and an increase in HDL, the "good" cholesterol, after following the low-carb diet (Westman et al., 2008). These success stories underscore the potential of low-carb living to transform health and well-being.

Dr. Westman offers practical advice to help you maintain a low-carb lifestyle. Meal planning and preparation are key. Start by creating a weekly meal plan that includes various low-carb foods to simplify grocery shopping and ensure you have healthy options readily available. Batch cooking can save time and make it easier to stick to your diet. Prepare large portions of low-carb meals and store them in the fridge or freezer for quick access (Westman, 2020).

Monitoring your progress is crucial for staying on track. Dr. Westman suggests keeping a food diary to record what you eat and how it affects your body. A diary can help you identify patterns and make necessary adjustments. Regularly check your weight, blood sugar levels, and other health markers to gauge your progress. If you hit a plateau or experience any issues, tweak your diet accordingly. Addressing common questions and misconceptions is also part of Dr. Westman's approach. For instance, many people worry about the impact of a low-carb diet on their cholesterol levels. Dr. Westman explains that while LDL cholesterol may initially rise, these LDL particles are usually large, fluffy particles that are not considered harmful. He also emphasizes the importance of looking at the overall lipid profile, including HDL and triglycerides, to get a complete picture of heart health (Westman et al., 2008).

Dr. Westman's approach to low-carb living is grounded in science, research, and practical experience. You can achieve significant health improvements by limiting carbohydrate intake, emphasizing whole foods, and ensuring a balance of protein and healthy fats. His clinical findings and patient success stories offer real-world evidence of the benefits of this lifestyle. With practical tips for meal planning, navigating social situations, and monitoring progress, Dr. Westman provides a comprehensive guide to adopting and maintaining a low-carb diet.

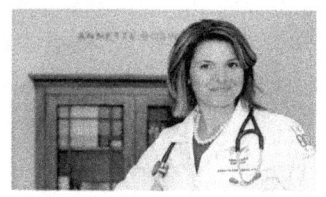

### 3.4 Dr. Annette Bosworth's Insights on Metabolic Health

Meet Dr. Annette Bosworth (Dr. Boz), a physician dedicated to unraveling the complexities of metabolic health and low-carb diets. With a medical degree and years of clinical experience, Dr. Bosworth has become an influential voice in the world of nutrition. Her journey with metabolic health began with personal struggles. Battling weight issues and low energy, she turned to low-carb diets as a solution (Bosworth, 2020). The dramatic improvements she experienced ignited her passion for metabolic health research. Dr. Bosworth has since contributed significantly to the field, sharing her insights through publications, public speaking, and patient consultations. Her book *KetoContinuum* lays out how Dr. Boz uses low-carb Keto to significantly improve her patients' health (Bosworth, 2020).

Dr. Bosworth emphasizes several critical concepts for achieving metabolic health. One of the most important is insulin sensitivity. Insulin is a hormone that helps regulate blood sugar levels. When your body becomes resistant to insulin, it struggles to manage glucose effectively, leading to conditions like type 2 diabetes (Mattson, Longo, & Harvie, 2017). Improving insulin sensitivity is critical to maintaining stable blood sugar levels and overall metabolic health. Dr. Bosworth advocates for dietary changes that enhance insulin sensitivity, such as reducing carbohydrate intake and focusing on nutrient-dense foods (Bosworth, 2020).

Another concept Dr. Bosworth highlights is intermittent fasting. This eating pattern involves cycling between periods of eating and fasting. It's not about what you eat but when you eat. Intermittent fasting can help improve insulin sensitivity, promote weight loss, and enhance metabolic health (Mattson et al., 2017). Dr. Bosworth often recommends starting with a simple fasting window, such as 16 hours of fasting followed by an 8-hour eating period. This approach allows your body to rest and repair, promoting better metabolic function (Bosworth, 2020).

Low-carb diets significantly influence Dr. Bosworth's approach to metabolic health. Dr. Bosworth emphasizes the importance of choosing whole, unprocessed foods rich in nutrients to ensure you get essential vitamins and minerals while keeping your carbohydrate intake low (Bosworth, 2020).

Lifestyle factors like sleep and stress also impact metabolic health. Dr. Bosworth stresses the importance of getting enough quality sleep. Poor sleep can disrupt your body's ability to regulate blood sugar and increase insulin resistance (Walker, 2017). She recommends creating a consistent sleep schedule, avoiding screens before bedtime, and creating a relaxing bedtime routine (Walker, 2017). Managing stress is equally important. Chronic stress can elevate cortisol levels, negatively affecting insulin sensitivity and metabolic health. Techniques like mindfulness meditation, deep breathing exercises, and regular physical activity can help reduce stress and improve overall well-being (Chrousos, 2009).

The health benefits Dr. Bosworth has observed through her practice and research are compelling. Improved blood sugar control is one of the most significant outcomes. Patients who adopt her recommendations often see their blood sugar levels stabilize, reducing the need for medication and lowering the risk of diabetes-related complications (Bosworth, 2020). Enhanced energy and vitality are other common benefits. By optimizing metabolic health, patients report feeling more energetic and capable of engaging in daily activities and exercise. Reducing the risk of chronic diseases is another critical benefit. Improved insulin sensitivity and lower blood sugar levels can decrease the risk of conditions like heart disease, stroke, and certain cancers (Mattson et al., 2017).

Focus on incorporating more nutrient-dense foods into your diet, such as leafy greens, lean proteins, and healthy fats. These foods provide essential nutrients without spiking your blood sugar levels. Incorporating intermittent fasting can also be beneficial. Start with a manageable fasting window and gradually increase it as your body adapts. This practice can help improve insulin sensitivity and support weight loss (Bosworth, 2020).

Regular health check-ups are crucial for monitoring your progress. Dr. Bosworth recommends tracking your blood sugar levels, weight, and other health markers to see how your body responds to dietary changes. Regular check-ups with your healthcare provider can help you make necessary adjustments and ensure you're on the right track. Monitoring your progress can also motivate you to stay committed to your new eating habits (Bosworth, 2020).

Dr. Bosworth's insights provide a valuable roadmap for improving metabolic health. Focusing on insulin sensitivity, incorporating intermittent fasting, and adopting a low-carb diet can enhance your energy levels, stabilize your blood sugar, and reduce the risk of chronic diseases. Her practical tips make it easier to navigate these changes and achieve better health.

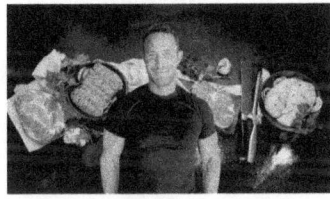

## 3.5 Dr. Anthony Chaffee's Nutritional Wisdom

Dr. Anthony Chaffee is a well-respected figure in the realm of nutrition, known for his extensive research and practical approach to dietary health. With a robust medical background, Dr. Chaffee has carved out a niche focusing on the profound impacts of nutrition on overall well-being. His credentials are impressive; he holds a medical degree and has spent years in clinical practice, seeing firsthand how dietary changes can transform health. Dr. Chaffee's journey with nutrition began with his personal health struggles. Battling issues like chronic fatigue and digestive problems, he turned to nutrition as a solution. This personal experience and his professional expertise have fueled his contributions to nutritional research, making him a trusted voice in the field (Chaffee, 2023).

Dr. Chaffee's nutritional philosophy is rooted in a whole-food focus. He believes that the most significant health benefits come from eating foods in their most natural state. He prioritizes foods that are minimally processed and rich in nutrients. Nutrient density is paramount. According to Dr. Chaffee, meats and seafood on the market today are the most nutrient-dense foods for us to consume daily (Chaffee, 2023).

One of Dr. Chaffee's more unique stances is his view on plants. He often says, "Plants are trying to kill you." While this statement is provocative, it underscores his belief that many plants contain toxins and anti-nutrients that can be harmful. He advocates for being mindful of plant consumption and focusing instead on nutrient-dense animal products. This approach aims to minimize the intake of potentially harmful substances while maximizing nutrient intake (Chaffee, 2023).

The health benefits observed by Dr. Chaffee in his patients are compelling. Enhanced immune function is one of the most notable improvements. Patients often experience fewer illnesses and a more robust immune system by eliminating processed foods and focusing on nutrient-dense options (Chaffee, 2023). Better mental clarity and cognitive function are also commonly reported. Nutrient-rich diets provide the brain with the essential nutrients to function optimally, improving focus, memory, and overall mental performance (Chaffee, 2023). Enhanced physical performance is another significant benefit. Patients often find that they have more energy and stamina, allowing them to engage in physical activities more effectively (Chaffee, 2023).

For those looking to adopt a healthier diet, Dr. Chaffee offers practical advice. Focus on incorporating more meats, eggs, seafood, and healthy fats into your meals. These foods provide essential nutrients without the harmful additives found in processed foods and plants (Chaffee, 2023).

Dr. Chaffee's insights provide a valuable framework for improving your health through nutrition. Focusing on whole, nutrient-dense foods and avoiding processed options can enhance your immune function, improve mental clarity, and boost physical performance. His practical advice makes it easier to navigate dietary changes and achieve lasting health benefits (Chaffee, 2023).

This chapter introduced various doctor-approved approaches to various diets and their unique benefits. Each expert offers a somewhat different approach, yet they all emphasize the importance of nutrition in achieving optimal health. You have also undoubtedly noticed how each of these healthcare professionals is similar in reducing carbohydrates in their approach to nutrition. Next, we will explore practical meal planning and how to make these dietary changes work for you daily.

# 4

# Practical Meal Planning: Making Diet Work for You

Imagine walking into your kitchen each morning, knowing exactly what you'll eat that day and how it fits into your health goals. Picture your confidence, knowing that preparing every meal supports your journey toward better health. This sense of control and assurance is precisely what a well-structured meal plan can offer. When you have a clear strategy, you're not just winging it; you're setting yourself up for success. A tailored meal plan ensures nutrient diversity, prevents deficiencies, and supports consistent energy levels, which are crucial for maintaining health and achieving your dietary goals (Harvard T.H. Chan School of Public Health, n.d.).

Creating a balanced meal plan starts with assessing your current dietary habits. Take a week to jot down everything you eat and drink. This food diary will give you a clear picture of your eating patterns and highlight areas that need improvement (Mayo Clinic, 2023). Are you consuming too many processed foods? Are your meals missing key nutrients like protein or healthy fats?

Identifying these gaps is the first step toward crafting a meal plan that works for you.

Next, set your dietary goals. What do you want to achieve? Are you aiming to lose weight, build muscle, improve your energy levels, or perhaps all three? Clear goals will guide your meal planning process. Once you have your goals, it's time to allocate your macronutrient ratios to determine how much of your diet will come from proteins, fats, and carbohydrates (Academy of Nutrition and Dietetics, 2023). For instance, if you're following a Keto diet, you'll allocate a higher percentage of your calories to fats and a lower percentage to carbs (Harvard Medical School, 2022). Tools like macronutrient calculators can help you determine the right balance to meet your goals.

The components of a tailored meal are straightforward but essential. Start with protein sources. Proteins are the building blocks of your body, crucial for muscle maintenance and repair (Harvard T.H. Chan School of Public Health, n.d.). Include ruminant meats, fish, eggs, and plant-based proteins like beans and lentils in your meals if you practice Paleo (Cordain, 2010). Healthy fats are another essential component. Saturated fats, once considered unhealthy, are now a staple in these diets. They provide a steady energy source and support brain health (Cleveland Clinic, 2023). Opt for fats from avocados, nuts, seeds, bacon grease, beef tallow, and olive oil. Keeping vegetables to a small part of your overall calories is essential in these diets. Vegetables with low-carb counts include leafy greens, broccoli, carrots, and bell peppers (Harvard Medical School, 2022).

### 4.1 Meal Planning Template and Practical Tips

Using a meal planning template can simplify the process. Start by sketching out your weekly meals, including breakfast, lunch, dinner, and snacks. This visual plan helps you see the variety and balance in your diet (Academy of Nutrition and Dietetics, 2023). Incorporating leftovers is another practical tip. Cooking larger portions and repurposing them for future meals saves time and ensures you always have healthy options. For instance, roast a whole chicken for dinner and use the leftovers in a salad or wrap the next day.

Creating a shopping list based on your meal plan is essential. A well-prepared list ensures you buy only the necessary foods, reducing food waste and saving money (Mayo Clinic, 2023). It also helps you avoid impulse buys, keeping you on track with your dietary goals. Organize your list by food categories—proteins, vegetables, fruits, dairy, and pantry staples—so shopping becomes more efficient. Also, consider this about nearly every modern grocery store: Eating a Ketogenic, Carnivore, or Paleo diet allows you to shop in a very small area of the store, as almost all of the whole foods you will be consuming are located around the perimeter of the store (Cordain, 2010). So take your list and only traverse through the produce, fruits and vegetables, meats, fish, and dairy sections to fill your cart in record time and leave all the junk food alone. Your wallet will also thank you for making this change.

Consider the example of planning a week's worth of balanced meals. For breakfast, you might start with scrambled eggs and spinach one day, followed by Greek yogurt with berries the next. These meals provide a mix of protein, healthy fats, and fiber to kickstart your day. Lunch could include a grilled chicken salad with various vegetables and a homemade vinaigrette. The next day, you might enjoy bacon and eggs, avocado, and a squeeze of lime. Dinners can be just as diverse—think baked salmon with asparagus one evening and a hearty beef stir-fry the next. Snacks can be simple yet nutritious: a handful of almonds, carrot sticks with hummus, or a piece of fruit on diets that allow these items (Harvard T.H. Chan School of Public Health, n.d.).

Adopting these practical tips and creating a tailored meal plan can transform your approach to eating. It's not just about what you eat but how you organize and prepare your meals. This structured approach ensures you get the necessary nutrients while making the process manageable and enjoyable (Academy of Nutrition and Dietetics, 2023). By taking control of your meal planning, you set yourself up for long-term success, making it easier to stick to your dietary goals and maintain a healthy lifestyle.

## 4.2 Nutrient-Dense Foods for Seniors

When discussing nutrient-dense foods, we're referring to foods packed with vitamins, minerals, and other essential nutrients but low in empty calories. These foods provide the building blocks your body needs to function optimally without processed foods' added sugars and unhealthy fats. For seniors, nutrient-dense foods are incredibly crucial. Your body requires more nutrients to maintain health and vitality, but your appetite and metabolism often slow as you age, so every bite you take should be rich in the nutrients that support overall health, from immune function to cognitive well-being (National Institute on Aging, 2021).

Let's start with some examples of nutrient-dense foods that you can easily incorporate into your diet. Fatty red meats, such as grass-fed beef, are excellent sources of protein, iron, and B vitamins. These nutrients are vital for muscle maintenance, energy production, and overall cellular health (Harvard T.H. Chan School of Public Health, n.d.). Berries, like blueberries and strawberries, are another fantastic option. They're loaded with antioxidants, vitamins, and fiber, all supporting immune function and digestive health (U.S. Department of Agriculture, 2020). Fatty fish, such as salmon and mackerel, provide omega-3 fatty acids essential for brain health and reducing inflammation (American Heart Association, 2019). Eggs are a versatile and nutrient-rich food, offering high-quality protein, vitamins A and D, and choline, which supports brain function (Mayo Clinic, 2022).

Incorporating these foods into your diet can bring about multiple health benefits. Improved immune function is one of the most immediate advantages. Nutrient-dense foods help strengthen your immune system, so you're less likely to fall ill and can recover more quickly when you do (National Institute on Aging, 2021). Enhanced cognitive health is another significant benefit. The omega-3s found in fatty fish and the choline in eggs are crucial for maintaining brain health (American Heart Association, 2019). These nutrients can improve memory, focus, and overall cognitive function, helping you stay sharp as you age (Harvard T.H. Chan School of Public Health, n.d.).

Better cardiovascular health is yet another benefit of eating nutrient-dense foods. Fatty fish like salmon and mackerel are rich in omega-3 fatty acids, which reduce the risk of heart disease by lowering blood pressure, reducing triglycerides, and preventing plaque buildup in the arteries (American Heart Association, 2019). With their high antioxidant content, berries help protect your heart by reducing oxidative stress and inflammation (U.S. Department of Agriculture, 2020). Grass-fed beef, when consumed in these diets, provides essential nutrients like iron and B vitamins that support heart health without the added saturated fats found in highly processed meats (Harvard T.H. Chan School of Public Health, n.d.).

Consider starting with simple recipes and snacks to make it easier to incorporate these foods into your diet. For example, a breakfast of scrambled eggs with spinach and a side of berries can provide a nutrient-packed start to your day. Lunch could be a salad topped with grilled salmon, avocado, and a sprinkle of nuts for added crunch and nutrients. For dinner, try a grass-fed beef stir-fry with various colorful vegetables. These meals are not only delicious but also ensure you get a balanced intake of vitamins, minerals, and other essential nutrients (Mayo Clinic, 2022).

Staying hydrated is also crucial for maintaining overall health, especially as you age. Drinking enough water can help with digestion, nutrient absorption, and keeping your skin healthy (National Institute on Aging, 2021). Herbal teas and infused water can be a great way to add variety to your hydration routine. For instance, adding slices of cucumber, lemon, or mint to your water can make it more enjoyable to drink and provide additional nutrients (Mayo Clinic, 2022).

Making these changes might seem overwhelming at first, but start small. Begin by incorporating one or two nutrient-dense foods into your daily meals, and gradually add more as you become comfortable. Your body will thank you for the extra nutrients, and you'll likely notice improvements in your energy levels, mental clarity, and overall well-being (U.S. Department of Agriculture, 2020).

As always, consult your healthcare provider before making significant changes to your diet, especially if you have existing health conditions or are taking medication. This way, you can tailor your diet to meet your specific needs and achieve the best possible outcomes for your health (Mayo Clinic, 2022).

## 4.3 Easy and Delicious Keto Recipes

Starting your day with a nutritious, keto-friendly breakfast can set the tone for the rest of your day. One of my favorite recipes is avocado and egg muffins. They're simple to make and packed with healthy fats and protein. Just mix some avocado with beaten eggs, cheese, and a pinch of salt and pepper. Pour the mixture into a muffin tin and bake until they're golden brown. These muffins are not only delicious but also convenient for busy mornings (Perfect Keto, 2022).

Another great option is a keto smoothie bowl. Blend some unsweetened almond milk, a handful of spinach, a scoop of protein powder, and a few berries. Pour the smoothie into a bowl and top it with nuts, seeds, and a drizzle of almond butter. This refreshing breakfast provides a good balance of protein, healthy fats, and fiber (Mayo Clinic, 2021). If you prefer something warm, try a cheese and spinach omelet. Whisk some eggs, add a handful of spinach and a sprinkle of your favorite cheese, and cook it in a skillet until the eggs are set. It's a hearty meal that will keep you satisfied all morning (Harvard T.H. Chan School of Public Health, n.d.).

For lunch, you can prepare a chicken Caesar salad with homemade dressing. Start with a bed of romaine lettuce, add some grilled chicken, and top it with Parmesan cheese and crispy bacon bits. Mix some Keto-friendly mayonnaise, lemon juice, Dijon mustard, and anchovy paste for the dressing. This salad is tasty and provides a good dose of protein and healthy fats (American Heart Association, 2020). Another quick option is zucchini noodles with pesto and grilled shrimp. Use a spiralizer to create zucchini noodles, sauté them in a bit of olive oil, and toss them with homemade or store-bought pesto. Top the noodles with grilled shrimp for a light yet satisfying meal (Harvard T.H. Chan School of Public Health, n.d.).

Another excellent lunch idea is keto-friendly wraps using lettuce leaves. Fill large lettuce leaves with your choice of protein, such as turkey or tuna, and add avocado slices, cucumber, and a dollop of Keto-friendly mayonnaise. These wraps are easy to prepare and perfect for a quick, low-carb lunch (Perfect Keto, 2022).

Dinner is the time to enjoy a hearty and satisfying meal. One of my go-to recipes is baked salmon with garlic butter. Season a salmon fillet with salt and pepper, place it on a baking sheet, and top it with a mixture of melted butter, minced garlic, and chopped parsley. Bake it until the salmon is cooked through and flaky. This dish is rich in omega-3 fatty acids and pairs well with a side of roasted vegetables (American Heart Association, 2020).

Beef stir-fry with low-carb vegetables is another delicious dinner option. Sauté thinly sliced beef in a hot skillet, then add your favorite low-carb vegetables, such as bell peppers, broccoli, and snap peas. Stir in a sauce made from coconut aminos, ginger, and garlic. This stir-fry is quick to prepare and full of flavor (Harvard T.H. Chan School of Public Health, n.d.). For a more indulgent meal, try making a cauliflower crust pizza. Pulse cauliflower florets in a food processor until they resemble rice, then mix them with an egg, some cheese, and seasonings. Press the mixture into a pizza crust shape and bake until crispy. Top with your favorite low-carb toppings, such as pepperoni, mushrooms, and mozzarella, and bake until the cheese is melted and bubbly (Mayo Clinic, 2021).

Snacks and desserts don't have to be off-limits on a keto diet. Keto fat bombs are a popular choice. These small, bite-sized treats are a mix of cream cheese, butter, and low-carb sweeteners and provide a quick energy boost (Perfect Keto, 2022). Almond flour cookies are another great option. Mix almond flour, a low-carb sweetener, and an egg to create a dough, then bake until golden brown. These cookies are perfect for satisfying your sweet tooth without derailing your diet (Mayo Clinic, 2021).

Cheese crisps are a savory snack that's easy to make. Simply place small mounds of shredded cheese on a baking sheet and bake until crispy and golden. They're a great alternative to chips and provide a satisfying crunch. These keto-friendly recipes make it easy to enjoy delicious and nutritious meals while sticking to your dietary goals. Whether you're preparing breakfast, lunch, dinner, or snacks, there are plenty of options that are both tasty and compliant with the keto diet (Harvard T.H. Chan School of Public Health, n.d.).

### 4.4 Simple Carnivore Meals

Starting your day with a hearty, carnivore-friendly breakfast can set a positive tone. Scrambled eggs with bacon is a classic that always works. Simply whisk the eggs, add a splash of cream, and cook them in a skillet with crispy bacon. This meal is delicious and provides a good mix of protein and healthy fats to keep you energized (Peterson, 2020). Another great breakfast option is steak and eggs. Season a steak with salt and pepper, cook it to your liking, and serve it alongside a couple of fried eggs. If you prefer something quick and easy, pork sausage patties are perfect. You can make a batch ahead of time and reheat them as needed. These patties are flavorful and packed with protein, making them an excellent start to your day (Carnivore Aurelius, 2022).

Lunchtime on the Carnivore diet doesn't have to be complicated. Grilled chicken thighs are a simple yet satisfying option. Season the chicken with salt, pepper, and your favorite herbs, then grill until the skin is crispy and the meat is cooked through. Serve it with a side of bone broth for added nutrients (Sisson, 2021). Beef liver pâté is another fantastic choice. While liver might not be everyone's favorite, it's incredibly nutrient-dense and offers a wealth of vitamins and minerals. To make the pâté, sauté liver with onions and garlic, then blend it until smooth. Spread it on slices of cooked bacon for a delicious and nutrient-packed lunch (Saladino, 2020).

Lamb chops are another easy and delicious lunch option. Season the chops with salt, pepper, and rosemary, then sear them in a hot skillet until done to your liking. The rich lamb flavor makes this a satisfying meal that doesn't require any sides (Peterson, 2020). You can also prepare a batch of pork belly bites for a quick and easy option. Cut the pork belly into bite-sized pieces, season with salt, and roast in the oven until crispy. These bites are perfect for a quick lunch or even as a snack (Sisson, 2021).

Dinner on the Carnivore diet can be both satisfying and nutritious. Roasted pork belly is a crowd-pleaser. Season the pork belly with salt and pepper, then roast it in the oven until the skin is crispy and the meat is tender. Serve it with a simple herb butter made from softened butter mixed with chopped herbs like rosemary and thyme (Saladino, 2020). Ribeye steak with butter is another dinner favorite. Season the steak with salt and pepper, sear it in a hot skillet, and finish it with a pat of butter. The butter melts over the steak, creating a rich and flavorful sauce (Carnivore Aurelius, 2022).

Baked cod with butter is a lighter dinner option that's still packed with flavor. Season the cod with salt and pepper, place it in a baking dish, and top it with pats of butter and lemon slices. Bake until the fish is flaky and tender (Sisson, 2021). Slow-cooked beef stew is perfect when you want a comforting and hearty meal. Brown chunks of beef in a skillet, then transfer them to a slow cooker. Add bone broth, garlic, and herbs, and let it cook on low for several hours until the beef is melt-in-your-mouth tender. This stew is rich, flavorful, and perfect for a satisfying dinner (Peterson, 2020).

Sourcing quality meats is helpful but optional for the Carnivore diet. Choosing grass-fed options is a great start but is often unrealistic for some budgets. When cost is a factor, buy the best quality meats you can afford. While grass-fed meats are higher in omega-3 fatty acids and antioxidants, which benefit your health, standard grocery store beef will still supply you with all the essential nutrients (Harvard T.H. Chan School of Public Health, n.d.). Buying in bulk can save you money and ensure you always have quality meat on hand. Look for deals at local butchers or consider joining a meat CSA (Community Supported Agriculture) program. The benefits of organ meats can't be overstated. Liver, kidneys, and heart are incredibly nutrient-dense and offer vitamins and minerals that are hard to find in other cuts of meat. Incorporating these into your diet can boost your nutrient intake (Saladino, 2020).

Finding local butchers can make a big difference in the meat quality. Local butchers often source their meat from nearby farms, ensuring it's fresh and responsibly raised. Building a relationship with your butcher can also lead to special deals and custom cuts tailored to your preferences. When selecting meats, look for freshness indicators like color and texture. Fresh meat should be firm to the touch and have a vibrant color. Lightly processed meats, such as air-dried or smoked options, can also be excellent choices for variety and convenience (Sisson, 2021).

Focusing on quality meats and simple preparation methods, the carnivore diet allows you to enjoy delicious and nutritious meals. Whether you're starting your day with a hearty breakfast, enjoying a satisfying lunch, or preparing a comforting dinner, these recipes and tips make it easy to stick to your dietary goals.

## 4.5 Paleo-Friendly Dishes

Starting your day with a nourishing breakfast that aligns with Paleo principles can set you on the right track. One of my favorite recipes is sweet potato hash with eggs. To prepare, simply dice sweet potatoes and sauté them with onions, bell peppers, and a touch of olive oil until they're tender and slightly caramelized. Crack a few eggs into the skillet and cook until they reach your desired doneness. This dish is rich in vitamins and provides a balanced mix of carbohydrates, protein, and healthy fats (Cordain, 2011).

Another excellent breakfast option is Paleo pancakes made with almond flour. Mix almond flour, eggs, a splash of almond milk, and a pinch of baking powder to create a batter. Cook the pancakes on a hot griddle until they're golden brown. These pancakes are fluffy, delicious, and grain-free, making them a perfect Paleo-friendly breakfast (Wolf, 2016). Try a fruit and nut breakfast bowl for a quick and satisfying option. Combine a variety of fresh fruits like berries, banana slices, and apple chunks with a handful of nuts and seeds. Add a dollop of coconut yogurt for extra creaminess. This bowl is refreshing and packed with essential nutrients to kickstart your day (Ballantyne, 2014).

When it comes to lunch, balance and satisfaction are key. A chicken and avocado salad is a simple yet flavorful choice. Start with a bed of mixed greens; add grilled chicken strips, avocado slices, cherry tomatoes, and cucumber. Drizzle with olive oil and lemon juice for a light but filling meal (Wolf, 2016). Another option is turkey lettuce wraps. Use large lettuce leaves as your wrap and fill them with slices of roasted turkey, avocado, shredded carrots, and a sprinkle of nuts for added crunch. These wraps are easy to prepare and perfect for a quick, nutritious lunch (Cordain, 2011).

A grilled vegetable platter with tahini sauce is another fantastic lunch idea. Grill various vegetables like zucchini, bell peppers, eggplant, and mushrooms until they're tender and slightly charred. Serve them with a homemade tahini sauce made from tahini paste, lemon juice, garlic, and a bit of water to thin it out. This dish is not only colorful and vibrant but also packed with fiber, vitamins, and minerals (Ballantyne, 2014).

For dinner, hearty and flavorful meals are essential to keep you satisfied. Baked chicken with rosemary and garlic is a classic that never disappoints. Season chicken pieces with salt, pepper, fresh rosemary, and minced garlic. Bake in the oven until the chicken is golden and cooked through. The aroma of rosemary and garlic will fill your kitchen, making this dish as delightful to smell as it is to eat (Wolf, 2016).

Beef and vegetable stir-fry is another excellent dinner option that's both quick and nutritious. Sauté beef strips in a hot skillet, then mix your favorite vegetables like broccoli, bell peppers, and snap peas. Stir in a sauce made from coconut aminos, ginger, and garlic. This stir-fry is bursting with flavor and provides a balanced mix of protein and vegetables (Cordain, 2011). Stuffed bell peppers with ground turkey are another great choice. Cut the tops off bell peppers and remove the seeds. Fill them with a mixture of cooked ground turkey, diced tomatoes, onions, and spices. Bake until the peppers are tender and the filling is done. This dish is hearty, nutritious, and perfect for a satisfying dinner (Ballantyne, 2014).

Snacks and desserts can also be Paleo-friendly and delicious. Mixed nuts and dried fruit make for an easy and portable snack. Choose a variety of nuts like almonds, walnuts, and cashews, and pair them with dried fruits like apricots, raisins, or cranberries. This combination provides a good mix of healthy fats and natural sugars to energize you between meals (Wolf, 2016). Coconut macaroons are a delightful dessert option that's both sweet and satisfying. Mix shredded coconut with egg whites and a touch of honey, then bake until golden brown. These macaroons are chewy, flavorful, and perfect for satisfying your sweet tooth (Ballantyne, 2014).

Baked apple slices with cinnamon are another simple yet delicious dessert. Slice apples and arrange them on a baking sheet. Sprinkle with cinnamon and bake until the apples are tender and caramelized. This dessert is warm, comforting, and naturally sweet without any added sugars (Cordain, 2011). These Paleo-friendly recipes make it easy to enjoy delicious and nutritious meals while sticking to your dietary principles. Whether you're preparing breakfast, lunch, dinner, or snacks, plenty of options are both tasty and compliant with the Paleo diet.

Now that we have explored these various unconventional diets, I hope you have picked one out and begun to improve your life. As you get healthier, you will be able to do more with your body, so let's look at how we can safely begin an exercise program. In the next chapter, we'll explore starting exercise routines, focusing on safely getting moving and building strength, balance, and flexibility.

## Make a Difference with Your Review

*"A healthy diet and regular exercise help you feel your best at any age. It's never too late to start."*

Dr. Eric Westman

People who take charge of their diet and exercise feel stronger, healthier, and happier. Let's make a difference together!

**Would you help someone just like you—curious about improving their health but unsure where to begin?**

My goal with *The Complete Beginner's Guide to Diet and Exercise for Seniors* is to make getting healthy easy and enjoyable for everyone. But to reach more people, I need your help.

Most people decide to read a book based on what others say about it. By leaving a review, you can help a fellow reader start their own journey to feeling great. And it only takes a minute!

Your review could mean so much:

- one more senior finds a path to better health.
- one more family member sees their loved one regain energy.
- one more community becomes healthier together.
- one more life transformed, and one more goal achieved.

To make a difference, simply scan below and leave a review:

If you love helping others, then you're my kind of person. Thank you from the bottom of my heart!

**Alex Silver**

# 5

# Starting an Exercise Routine: Getting Moving Safely

Think about Jane, a 70-year-old woman who always believed that her aches and pains were simply a part of aging. One day, she decided enough was enough. Jane realized that she needed to start moving more to improve her quality of life. But where to begin? Jane did not know her current fitness level and feared overexerting herself and risking injury. That's why Jane learned to assess her fitness level before jumping into an exercise routine.

## 5.1 Assessing Your Current Fitness Level

Before you lace up your sneakers and start exercising, it's crucial to understand your starting point. Assessing your fitness level helps establish a baseline, identify strengths and weaknesses, and tailor exercise plans to your specific needs. This process is essential for setting realistic goals and avoiding injury. Knowing where you stand allows you to measure progress and stay motivated. It's like setting out on a road trip with a map; you need to know your starting location to plan your route effectively (Centers for Disease Control and Prevention [CDC], 2022).

Establishing this baseline is the first step, which involves taking note of your current physical abilities, such as how long you can walk without feeling breathless or how many times you can stand up from a chair without using your hands. This initial assessment provides a snapshot of your fitness and a foundation upon which to build (American Heart Association [AHA], 2021). It's also a great way to identify areas that need improvement, whether cardiovascular endurance, muscle strength, or flexibility. Tailoring your exercise plan based on these insights ensures that you're working on areas that will benefit you the most, making your efforts more effective and rewarding (American College of Sports Medicine [ACSM], 2021).

For a simple self-assessment, you can start with basic cardiovascular tests, strength tests, and flexibility tests. For cardiovascular fitness, try a walking test. Measure how long you can walk at a steady pace without feeling overly tired. Note any discomfort or breathlessness. Strength tests can include the chair sit-to-stand exercise. Sit in a sturdy chair and stand up without using your hands. Repeat this as many times as you can within a minute. This test helps measure lower body strength and endurance (ACSM, 2021). Flexibility tests such as the sit-and-reach can provide insights into your range of motion. Sit on the floor with your legs straight and try to reach your toes. Note how far you can go without straining. These simple tests provide valuable information about your fitness level and highlight areas needing attention (CDC, 2022).

While self-assessment is a valuable starting point, seeking professional help for a comprehensive fitness evaluation can offer more detailed insights. Consulting a physical therapist is particularly beneficial if you have existing health conditions or concerns about injury. A physical therapist can conduct a thorough assessment, considering your medical history and specific needs. They can also provide personalized recommendations and modifications to ensure your exercise routine is safe and effective (Mayo Clinic, 2021). Understanding health conditions is another crucial aspect. Certain conditions, like arthritis or heart disease, may require specific precautions or adaptations in your exercise plan. A professional assessment ensures that these factors are considered, reducing the risk of complications and enhancing the benefits of your exercise regimen (AHA, 2021).

To help you get started, here's a fitness assessment checklist that you can use to record your assessments. Begin with heart rate measurements. Take your pulse before and after physical activities to see how your heart responds to exercise. Note the duration of physical activities, such as how long you can walk or perform a particular exercise without feeling overly fatigued. Pay attention to your mobility and range of motion. Record how far you can stretch or how easily you can move your joints. This checklist helps track your progress over time and provides a clear picture of your fitness journey (ACSM, 2021).

**Fitness Assessment Checklist:**

- Heart Rate Measurements: Take your pulse before and after physical activities.
- Duration of Physical Activities: Note how long you can walk or perform exercises without fatigue.
- Mobility and Range of Motion: Record how far you can stretch and the ease of joint movements.

Assessing your fitness level is a crucial step in starting an exercise routine. It provides a clear understanding of your starting point, helps set realistic goals, and ensures that your exercise plan meets your needs. Whether through self-assessment or professional evaluation, taking the time to understand your fitness level will set you up for success and reduce the risk of injury (Mayo Clinic, 2021).

## 5.2 Warm-Up and Cool-Down Exercises

You wouldn't start your car on a cold winter morning and immediately speed off without letting it warm up a bit, would you? The same principle applies to your body. Warming up before exercising is crucial because it prepares your muscles and cardiovascular system for the work ahead. Think of it as gently waking up your body. Engaging in warm-up exercises increases blood flow to your muscles, which helps deliver the oxygen and nutrients they need (American College of Sports Medicine [ACSM], 2021). This increased circulation also raises your muscle temperature, making them more pliable and less prone to injury. Warm-up exercises enhance muscle flexibility, allowing for a greater range of motion and reducing the risk of strains and sprains (Mayo Clinic, 2021).

A practical warm-up routine doesn't have to be complicated. Gentle marching in place is an excellent starting point. It gets your heart rate up slightly and starts the process of warming your leg muscles. Arm circles are another great option. Extend your arms out to your sides and make small, controlled circles, gradually increasing the size. This helps loosen up your shoulder joints and improves blood flow to your upper body. Leg swings are also effective. Stand next to a wall for balance and gently swing one leg forward and backward, then switch to the other leg. This movement helps mobilize your hip joints and stretches your leg muscles (ACSM, 2021). Lastly, neck rotations can be very beneficial. Slowly turn your head from side to side and then up and down, which helps release tension in your neck and prepares your cervical spine for activity (Harvard Health Publishing, 2020).

Just as important as warming up is cooling down after your workout. Cooling down helps your body transition back to a resting state. One of the primary benefits is gradually lowering your heart rate. When you suddenly stop exercising, your heart rate can drop too quickly, leading to dizziness or lightheadedness. A proper cool-down routine helps prevent this by allowing your heart rate to decrease slowly and steadily (Mayo Clinic, 2021). Another benefit is reducing muscle stiffness. After a workout, your muscles can tighten up, leading to soreness. Cooling down helps relax your muscles and reduces the buildup of lactic acid, which can contribute to muscle stiffness (ACSM, 2021). Additionally, cooling down can help prevent dizziness and fainting, which can occur if blood pools in your lower extremities and doesn't return to your heart efficiently (Harvard Health Publishing, 2020).

A cool-down routine should include gentle stretching and deep breathing exercises. Begin with gentle stretching to help your muscles relax and elongate. For example, you can do a simple hamstring stretch by sitting on the floor with your legs extended in front of you and reaching for your toes. Hold the stretch for 10-20 seconds without bouncing. Deep breathing exercises are also beneficial. Inhale deeply through your nose, hold for a few seconds, and then exhale slowly through your mouth, which helps oxygenate your muscles and promotes relaxation (ACSM, 2021). Slow walking is another excellent cool-down activity. Walk leisurely for about five minutes to help your heart rate gradually return to normal. Static stretches for major muscle groups, like your calves, quadriceps, shoulders, and back, can also be very effective. Hold each stretch for 10-20 seconds, focusing on your breathing and allowing your muscles to relax fully (Mayo Clinic, 2021).

Incorporating a proper warm-up and cool-down routine into your exercise regimen is vital to maintaining a safe and effective workout program. By preparing your body for physical activity and helping it recover afterward, you reduce the risk of injury, enhance muscle flexibility, and ensure that your workouts are as beneficial as possible. These routines don't have to be lengthy or complicated, but their impact on your overall fitness and well-being can be profound.

### 5.3 Walking for Health: The Easiest Exercise

Walking is an ideal exercise for seniors for many reasons. First, it's a low-impact activity, which means it's easy on your joints and less likely to cause injury than high-impact exercises like running. Therefore, walking is accessible for almost anyone, regardless of fitness level. Moreover, walking is fantastic for improving cardiovascular health. It helps strengthen your heart, lower blood pressure, and improve circulation (American Heart Association [AHA], 2021). Regular walking can significantly reduce the risk of heart disease and stroke, making it a crucial part of a healthy lifestyle. Beyond physical benefits, walking also enhances mood and mental health. The simple act of getting outside, breathing fresh air, and moving your body can help reduce stress, anxiety, and symptoms of depression. Walking releases endorphins, the body's natural mood lifters, which can make you happier and more relaxed (Harvard Health Publishing, 2020). Additionally, walking is accessible and free. You don't need a gym membership or expensive equipment—just a good pair of shoes and a safe place to walk (AHA, 2021).

Starting a walking routine begins with choosing the right footwear. Proper shoes provide the support and cushioning your feet need to prevent discomfort and injury. Look for shoes specifically designed for walking, with good arch support and a comfortable fit. It's also important to find safe walking routes. Choose well-lit areas with smooth, even surfaces to reduce the risk of falls. Parks, walking trails, and quiet neighborhood streets are excellent options (Mayo Clinic, 2021). Setting walking goals can help you stay motivated and track your progress. Start with small, achievable goals, such as walking for 10 minutes daily, and gradually increase the duration. Incorporating walking into daily activities is another great strategy. Walk to the store instead of driving, take the stairs instead of the elevator, or enjoy a stroll around the block after dinner. These small changes can add up and make a big difference in your overall health (Harvard Health Publishing, 2020).

As you become more comfortable with your walking routine, you can gradually increase the intensity to continue challenging your body. One way to do this is by increasing the duration of your walks. If you start with 10 minutes a day, add 5 minutes each week until you walk for at least 30 minutes daily. Adding intervals of brisk walking can also boost the intensity. Try alternating between a moderate and a faster pace every few minutes, increasing your heart rate and improving cardiovascular fitness (AHA, 2021). Walking on varied terrains, such as hills or uneven paths, can engage different muscle groups and add an extra challenge. If you're looking for even more intensity, consider using walking poles. They provide additional support and help engage your upper body, turning your walk into a full-body workout (Mayo Clinic, 2021).

Here's a sample walking plan to help you start and gradually increase your walking duration. In Week 1, aim to walk for 10 minutes daily. Focus on getting comfortable with the routine and ensuring you have the proper footwear and a safe route. In Week 2, increase your walking time to 15 minutes each day. By now, you should start feeling more confident and may already notice some benefits, such as improved mood and increased energy. In Week 3, extend your walks to 20 minutes daily. You can start experimenting with different routes or incorporate some intervals of brisk walking. Finally, in Week 4, aim for 25 minutes of walking each day. By the end of this month, you'll have established a solid walking routine that you can continue to build on (AHA, 2021).

Walking is a simple yet powerful exercise that offers numerous benefits for seniors. It's low-impact, improves cardiovascular health, enhances mood, and is accessible and free. By choosing the right footwear, finding safe walking routes, setting achievable goals, and gradually increasing the intensity, you can make walking a regular part of your healthy lifestyle. So, grab your shoes, head outside, and start walking your way to better health.

### 5.4 Chair Exercises: Staying Active with Limited Mobility

Chair exercises are a fantastic way to stay active, especially with limited mobility. These exercises allow you to engage your muscles and improve your fitness without the strain that more demanding activities might cause. Sitting in a chair provides the stability and support you need, which is particularly useful if you have balance issues or joint pain. Chair exercises are suitable for all fitness levels, making them an excellent option whether you're a beginner or looking to supplement your existing routine (Mayo Clinic, 2021).

Let's look at some specific chair exercises that can help you get started. Seated leg lifts are a great way to strengthen your lower body. Sit upright in a sturdy chair with your feet flat on the floor. Slowly lift one leg, keeping it straight, and hold for a few seconds before lowering it back down. Repeat with the other leg. This exercise targets your quadriceps and can help improve leg strength and mobility (American College of Sports Medicine [ACSM], 2021). Arm raises with light weights are another effective exercise. Hold a light weight in each hand and sit with your back straight. Raise your arms to shoulder height, hold for a moment, and then lower them back down. This movement works your shoulder muscles and helps improve upper body strength (ACSM, 2021).

Seated marches are excellent for engaging your core and lower body. Sit tall in your chair and lift one knee towards your chest, then lower it and repeat with the other knee. Continue alternating for a set number of repetitions. This exercise mimics the motion of marching and can help improve your cardiovascular health and core strength (Mayo Clinic, 2021). Seated twists are perfect for working your obliques and improving spinal mobility. Sit with your feet flat on the floor and your back straight. Place your hands behind your head and gently twist your torso to one side, then return to the center and twist to the other side. This exercise helps enhance flexibility and core strength (Harvard Health Publishing, 2020).

Incorporating chair exercises into your fitness routine offers numerous benefits. Improved circulation is one of the primary advantages. Regular movement helps increase blood flow, reducing the risk of blood clots and improving overall cardiovascular health. Enhanced muscle strength is another significant benefit. Even simple exercises like leg lifts and arm raises can help build muscle mass, which is crucial for maintaining mobility and independence as you age (ACSM, 2021). Increased flexibility is also a key outcome. Exercises like seated twists and stretches help keep your joints and muscles flexible, reducing the risk of stiffness and injury (Harvard Health Publishing, 2020). Better balance and coordination are additional benefits, making everyday activities easier and safer (Mayo Clinic, 2021).

Here's a sample chair exercise routine to help you get started. Begin with a warm-up to prepare your muscles and get your blood flowing. Seated shoulder rolls are an excellent warm-up exercise. Sit straight and gently roll your shoulders forward and backward for a minute. This movement helps loosen up your shoulder joints and muscles. For the main exercises, aim for 10 repetitions of each. Start with seated leg lifts, followed by arm raises with light weights. Next, do seated marches, lifting each knee towards your chest, and then move on to seated twists, gently twisting your torso from side to side. These exercises target different muscle groups and provide a balanced workout. Finish with a cool-down to help your body recover. Gentle seated stretches are perfect for this. Stretch your arms, legs, and back while focusing on deep, slow breaths. Hold each stretch for 10-20 seconds, allowing your muscles to relax and elongate (ACSM, 2021).

Chair exercises are an excellent way to stay active and improve your fitness, even with limited mobility. They provide the stability and support you need while offering numerous benefits, such as improved circulation, enhanced muscle strength, increased flexibility, and better balance and coordination. By incorporating a variety of chair exercises into your routine, you can enjoy a well-rounded workout that supports your overall health and well-being. So, find a sturdy chair, set aside some time each day, and start exploring the many benefits of chair exercises.

## 5.5 Flexibility and Stretching: Preventing Stiffness

Flexibility is often overlooked but is crucial in maintaining an active and healthy lifestyle, especially as we age. Think about the ease of reaching for something on a high shelf or bending down to tie your shoes. These seemingly simple tasks require a good range of motion directly tied to your flexibility. Maintaining flexibility helps reduce the risk of injury by allowing your muscles and joints to move freely and efficiently (Harvard Health Publishing, 2020). When your muscles are flexible, they can stretch and contract without causing damage, reducing the likelihood of strains or sprains during daily activities or exercise. Improved flexibility also enhances your range of motion, making it easier to perform tasks that involve bending, stretching, or twisting. Flexibility leads to better functional movements, allowing you to move more freely and confidently in your daily life (ACSM, 2021).

Incorporating specific stretching exercises into your routine can significantly benefit your flexibility and overall mobility. Hamstring stretches are particularly effective for maintaining flexibility in your legs. Sit on the edge of a sturdy chair with one leg extended straight and the other foot flat on the floor. Reach forward towards your toes, keeping your back straight. Hold the stretch for 15-30 seconds without bouncing, then switch legs. Calf stretches are another excellent option. Stand facing a wall with one foot forward and the other foot back, keeping your back heel on the ground. Lean into the wall until you feel a stretch in your calf, hold for 10-20 seconds, and switch legs (Mayo Clinic, 2021). Shoulder stretches can help maintain upper body flexibility. Bring one arm across your chest and use your opposite hand to gently pull it closer. Hold the stretch for 10-20 seconds and repeat with the other arm. Hip flexor stretches are also beneficial. Kneel on one knee with the other foot in front, forming a 90-degree angle. Push your hips forward gently until you feel a stretch in your hip, hold for 10-20 seconds, and switch sides (ACSM, 2021).

Making stretching a part of your daily routine is easier than you think. Start by incorporating stretches into your morning routine. When you wake up, take a few minutes to perform simple stretches to loosen up your muscles and prepare your body for the day ahead. Stretching can be as simple as a few hamstring and calf stretches while you brush your teeth or make your bed. Another great time to stretch is during TV time. Instead of sitting on the couch for long periods, use commercial breaks or the beginning of your favorite show as a reminder to get up and stretch to maintain flexibility and break up long periods of inactivity (Harvard Health Publishing, 2020). You can also use stretching as a break during sedentary activities, such as working at a desk or reading. Set a timer to remind yourself to get up every 30 minutes and perform a quick stretch. These small changes can make a big difference in your overall flexibility and mobility (Mayo Clinic, 2021).

When it comes to stretching, safety is paramount. Avoid bouncing or jerky movements, which can cause muscle strains or tears. Instead, aim for smooth, controlled motions. Hold each stretch for 10-20 seconds, allowing your muscles to relax and elongate. Focus on your breathing while stretching. Inhale deeply through your nose and exhale slowly through your mouth. Breathing this way helps oxygenate your muscles and promotes relaxation (ACSM, 2021). Stretch both sides of your body equally to maintain balance and prevent muscle imbalances. For example, if you stretch your right hamstring, make sure to do the same for your left (Harvard Health Publishing, 2020).

Flexibility and stretching are vital components of a well-rounded fitness routine. Maintaining flexibility reduces the risk of injury, enhances your range of motion, and improves your daily functional movements. Incorporating effective stretching exercises like hamstring, calf, shoulder, and hip flexor stretches into your daily routine can help you stay agile and mobile. Remember to stretch in the morning, during TV time, and as breaks during sedentary activities. Follow safe stretching guidelines to get the most benefit without risking injury (Mayo Clinic, 2021).

Integrating stretching and flexibility exercises into your routine lays a solid foundation for a healthier, more active lifestyle. These practices enhance your physical capabilities and contribute to your overall well-being. In the next chapter, we'll explore balance and stability exercises, focusing on preventing falls and injuries and further supporting your journey toward better health.

# 6

# Balance and Stability: Preventing Falls and Injuries

Imagine the case of Carol, a vibrant 72-year-old who cherished her routine strolls through the local park. These walks were not just exercise; they were her daily dose of joy, connecting with nature and her community. But recently, Carol began to notice a troubling change: her steps felt uncertain, and her balance was precarious. Then, on a seemingly ordinary day, her fears materialized. While navigating an uneven patch of the pathway, she lost her footing and fell, sustaining a painful wrist fracture. This incident, more than just a physical setback, struck a blow to her confidence. The fall instilled a newfound apprehension toward engaging in her beloved walks. Carol's experience highlights the indispensable role of balance and stability as we navigate our senior years. It's a stark reminder that maintaining balance is about more than preventing falls; it's about preserving our autonomy, ensuring we can continue to embrace life's simple pleasures with assurance and vitality.

## 6.1 Understanding the Importance of Balance

Balance is crucial for seniors because it significantly reduces the risk of falls, a leading cause of injury among older adults. According to the Centers for Disease Control and Prevention (CDC), over 14 million older adults report falling each year, and about 37% of those falls result in injuries that require medical treatment or restrict activity for at least one day (CDC, 2023). These statistics highlight the urgency of addressing balance issues to prevent falls and their associated consequences. Good balance enhances your ability to move confidently and safely, whether walking on uneven surfaces, climbing stairs, or simply getting up from a chair.

Balance also supports mobility, making navigating your environment and performing daily activities easier. Imagine walking through a crowded room or an outdoor market without worrying about tripping or losing your footing. Improved balance means you can enjoy these activities more efficiently and less fearfully. It also supports independence, allowing you to live more freely without relying on others for assistance. When you can move confidently, you're more likely to engage in physical activities, socialize, and maintain a higher quality of life (Johns Hopkins Medicine, 2021).

Good balance reduces the risk of falls and prevents injuries. Falls often lead to severe injuries, such as hip fractures, which can be particularly debilitating for seniors. According to Johns Hopkins Medicine, falls can result from various factors, including vision changes, vestibular issues, and altered foot sensation (Johns Hopkins Medicine, 2021). These factors can make simple activities like getting up from the toilet or moving in a dark bedroom risky. You can mitigate these risks and protect yourself from injuries by improving your balance.

Several common causes contribute to poor balance in seniors. Muscle weakness is a significant factor. Muscle mass decreases naturally as we age unless we do something about it. Muscle loss affects our strength, stability, and ability to perform even simple tasks. Joint stiffness can also impair balance, making it harder to move fluidly and react quickly to changes in terrain or posture (American College of Sports Medicine [ACSM], 2021). Vision problems, such as cataracts or glaucoma, can affect depth perception and spatial awareness, increasing the risk of missteps and falls. Medication side effects are another consideration. Many seniors take multiple medications, which can cause dizziness or drowsiness, further compromising balance (CDC, 2023).

The impact of good balance on daily activities cannot be overstated. Walking on uneven surfaces becomes less daunting when your balance is strong. Whether navigating a gravel path or a grassy field, good balance helps you stay steady. Climbing stairs, a common challenge for many seniors, becomes more manageable with improved balance. You'll find lifting your feet easier and maintaining your stability as you ascend or descend. Getting in and out of chairs, a daily activity that requires strength and balance, becomes smoother and safer (ACSM, 2021).

Good balance also benefits reaching for objects, whether on high shelves or low cupboards. You'll feel more confident extending your arms and shifting your weight without the fear of toppling over. These daily activities improve your overall quality of life, allowing you to maintain your independence and enjoy a more active lifestyle.

Statistics on falls among seniors are sobering, as over 25% of adults aged 65 or older experience a fall each year, resulting in an estimated nine million fall injuries annually (CDC, 2023). The age-adjusted fall death rate has increased by 41% from 2012 to 2021, emphasizing the growing concern over fall-related injuries and fatalities. The highest fall death rate in 2021 was 176.5 per 100,000 in Wisconsin, illustrating the significant variability in fall rates across different states. These numbers highlight the critical need for fall prevention measures, including balance exercises and interventions to address risk factors (CDC, 2023).

The consequences of falls extend beyond physical injuries. They often lead to a loss of confidence, making seniors more fearful of engaging in physical activities. This fear can decrease mobility, further weaken muscles, and exacerbate balance issues. The financial costs of fall-related injuries are also substantial, including medical treatments, rehabilitation, and potential long-term care needs.

Understanding the importance of balance and taking proactive steps to improve it can significantly enhance your quality of life. Addressing the common causes of poor balance and incorporating balance exercises into your routine can reduce your risk of falls, improve your mobility, and maintain your independence. Balance is not just about avoiding falls; it's about living confidently and thoroughly enjoying your daily activities.

## 6.2 Simple Balance Exercises for Daily Practice

Improving your balance doesn't require complex routines or expensive equipment. Simple exercises can make a big difference, and you can easily fit them into your daily routine. Let's start with standing on one foot. This exercise is straightforward but highly effective. Begin by standing near a wall or a chair for support. Lift one foot off the ground and hold the position for as long as possible, aiming for at least 10 seconds. Switch to the other foot and repeat. Try to hold the position for longer periods as you get more comfortable. Clear starting positions and maintaining focus are crucial. Keep your gaze fixed on a point before you to help maintain your balance (American College of Sports Medicine [ACSM], 2021).

Another excellent exercise is the heel-to-toe walk. This activity improves your balance by challenging your coordination. Start by standing upright with your feet together. Take a step forward, placing the heel of one foot directly in front of the toes of the other foot. Continue walking in a straight line, placing each foot heel-to-toe. If you feel unsteady, use a wall or a handrail for support. Aim to walk this way for about 20 steps. This exercise enhances your balance and improves your gait, making walking easier and safer (Mayo Clinic, 2021).

Side leg raises are another simple yet effective exercise. Stand next to a sturdy chair or countertop for support. Slowly lift one leg out to the side, keeping it straight. Hold this position for a few seconds before lowering your leg back down. Repeat 10 times on each side. This exercise strengthens your hip muscles, which are crucial in maintaining balance. Keep your back straight and avoid leaning to the side, as this will help you engage the right muscles and benefit most from the exercise (Harvard Health Publishing, 2020).

Backward walking might seem unusual, but improving your balance and coordination is possible using this method. Find a safe, flat area where you can walk backward without obstacles. Begin by taking small steps backward, focusing on placing each foot carefully. Use a wall or handrail for support if needed. Walk backward for about 10 steps, then walk forward to your starting point. This exercise challenges your balance differently and helps improve your overall stability. It also engages different muscle groups, providing a well-rounded balance workout (ACSM, 2021).

Consistent practice of these balance exercises can significantly improve your stability. Gradual improvement is the key. Over time, you'll feel more stable and confident in your movements. This increased confidence can make a big difference in your daily life, whether walking through a crowded room or navigating uneven terrain. Enhanced coordination is another benefit of regular balance practice. As you challenge your body with these exercises, you'll develop better control over your movements, reducing the risk of falls and injuries.

As you become more comfortable with these exercises, you can increase the difficulty as you continue to challenge your balance. One way to do this is by closing your eyes while balancing, which removes visual cues and forces your body to rely on other senses, such as proprioception and inner ear balance. Start by standing on one foot with your eyes open, then close your eyes and try to maintain your balance. This exercise is more challenging, so ensure you have a wall or chair nearby for support (Mayo Clinic, 2021).

Adding light weights can also increase the difficulty of your balance exercises. For instance, you can hold small dumbbells while doing side leg raises or heel-to-toe walks. The added weight will engage your muscles more, providing a greater challenge and helping to build strength. Start with light weights and gradually increase as you get stronger (Harvard Health Publishing, 2020).

Performing exercises on an unstable surface, like a balance pad or a folded towel, can further enhance your balance training. The unstable surface forces your body to work harder to maintain stability, engaging more muscles and improving your overall balance. Start with simple exercises like standing on one foot or doing side leg raises on the balance pad. As you get more comfortable, you can try more challenging exercises (ACSM, 2021).

Increasing the duration of your balance exercises is another way to keep improving. For example, if you initially held the standing on one-foot position for 10 seconds, aim to increase it to 20 or 30 seconds. Gradually increasing the duration will continue to challenge your balance and help you make progress.

### 6.3 Tai Chi for Seniors: Improving Balance and Flexibility

Tai Chi, an ancient Chinese martial art, has found its way into the lives of seniors worldwide. It's not about high-impact moves or strenuous workouts; Tai Chi focuses on slow, deliberate movements and a solid mind-body connection. Originating centuries ago, Tai Chi began as a form of self-defense, but it has evolved into a practice cherished for its health benefits. The graceful, flowing movements help to circulate energy throughout the body, promoting balance and harmony. This harmony makes Tai Chi especially beneficial for seniors looking to improve their balance and flexibility (Wayne & Kaptchuk, 2008).

For seniors, Tai Chi offers a multitude of advantages. One of the most significant benefits is improved balance and coordination. The slow, controlled movements help enhance your body's awareness and stability, which is particularly important as we age, given the increased risk of falls. According to a scoping review by the National Institutes of Health, Tai Chi significantly improves balance, cardiorespiratory fitness, cognition, mobility, proprioception, sleep, and strength in older adults (Rogers et al., 2017). The practice also increases muscle strength, which is crucial for maintaining an active lifestyle. The gentle resistance of the movements helps build muscle without putting undue strain on the joints.

Another key benefit of Tai Chi is enhanced flexibility. The movements involve a full range of motion, which helps keep your joints fluid and flexible. Increased flexibility can be particularly beneficial for those with arthritis or joint stiffness (Harvard Health Publishing, 2020). Tai Chi also reduces stress and anxiety.

Focusing on deep breathing and mindful movement creates a meditative state, helping lower stress levels and promote a sense of calm. This holistic approach addresses both physical and mental well-being, making Tai Chi a comprehensive practice for seniors.

Let's explore a few simple Tai Chi movements that you can start practicing today. The "Commencement of Tai Chi" is often the first movement in many Tai Chi routines. Stand with your feet shoulder-width apart and your arms hanging naturally at your sides. Slowly raise your arms to shoulder height, palms facing downward, while bending your knees slightly. Then, lower your arms back to the starting position as you straighten your knees. This movement sets the tone for the practice, helping you focus and center yourself (Wayne & Kaptchuk, 2008).

Another foundational movement is "Parting the Horse's Mane." Begin with your feet shoulder-width apart and your arms relaxed. Step forward with your left foot while simultaneously raising your left arm in front of you and your right arm behind you as if you're holding a ball. Shift your weight onto your left foot, and then step forward with your right foot, switching the position of your arms. This movement mimics the action of parting a horse's mane and helps improve coordination and balance.

"Grasping the Bird's Tail" is a classic Tai Chi movement that combines several smaller movements into one fluid sequence. Start with your feet shoulder-width apart and your arms at your sides. Step forward with your left foot and raise your left arm to shoulder height, palm facing outward. Your right arm should be bent at the elbow, palm facing your chest. Shift your weight onto your left foot, and then step forward with your right foot. Extend your right arm forward and pull your left arm back as if grasping a bird's tail. This movement helps improve balance, coordination, and flexibility.

Starting Tai Chi can be an enriching experience, but it's essential to approach it mindfully. Finding a local class or online tutorial can guide you in getting started. Many community centers and senior organizations offer Tai Chi classes specifically designed for older adults. These classes provide a supportive environment where you can learn the movements at your own pace. If you prefer practicing at home, numerous online tutorials and videos can guide you through the basics (Rogers et al., 2017).

Wearing comfortable clothing is crucial. Choose loose-fitting, breathable clothes that allow you to move freely. Tai Chi involves a lot of stretching and bending, so you'll want to ensure your clothing doesn't restrict your movements. Practicing in a quiet, spacious area can enhance your experience. Find a spot in your home or garden where you won't be disturbed so you focus on your practice and fully engage in the movements.

Listening to your body and moving at a comfortable pace is essential. Tai Chi is not about pushing yourself to the limit but finding a rhythm that feels natural and sustainable. Pay attention to how your body feels and make adjustments as needed. If a movement feels uncomfortable or causes pain, modify it or skip it altogether. The goal is to create a practice that supports your well-being and brings you joy.

Tai Chi is a gentle yet powerful practice that significantly improves balance, flexibility, and overall well-being. With its focus on slow, deliberate movements and a strong mind-body connection, Tai Chi offers a holistic approach to health accessible to seniors of all fitness levels. Whether you join a class or practice at home, Tai Chi can become a cherished part of your daily routine, supporting your journey toward a more balanced and fulfilling life.

### 6.4 Yoga for Balance: Poses and Practices

Yoga, an ancient Indian practice, offers a blend of postures, breath control, and meditation. It's adaptable for all fitness levels, making it an excellent choice for seniors. Yoga emphasizes controlled movements and deep breathing, which can help you stay centered and focused. This practice is not just about physical flexibility; it's about enhancing your overall well-being. Whether you're new to yoga or have practiced it before, it brings many benefits, especially for balance (Harvard Health Publishing, 2021).

One of the standout benefits of yoga is enhanced body awareness. You develop a keen sense of balance by focusing on how your body moves and feels in different postures. Heightening your awareness helps you make small adjustments to maintain stability, reducing your risk of falls. Yoga also strengthens your core muscles, which are essential for good balance. A strong core supports your spine and helps you maintain proper posture, making everyday activities easier and safer (American College of Sports Medicine [ACSM], 2021).

Flexibility is another crucial benefit of yoga. Many seniors struggle with joint stiffness and limited range of motion. Yoga poses gently stretch your muscles and joints, improving flexibility and reducing discomfort. This increased flexibility makes it easier to move freely and perform daily tasks. Additionally, yoga is a powerful stress reducer. Combining physical movement, deep breathing, and meditation helps lower stress levels and promotes a sense of calm. This holistic approach to health can improve your mental well-being and make you feel more at ease in your body (Mayo Clinic, 2020).

Let's explore some yoga poses that are particularly effective for improving balance. The Tree Pose, or Vrksasana, is a great place to start. Stand with your feet together and shift your weight onto your left foot. Slowly lift your right foot and place it on your left inner thigh or calf, avoiding the knee. Bring your hands together in front of your chest, or raise them above your head. Focus on a point in front of you to maintain balance. Hold the pose for 20-30 seconds, then switch sides. This pose strengthens your legs and improves your focus and balance (Iyengar, 2001).

Warrior III, or Virabhadrasana III, is another excellent balance pose. Stand with your feet together and shift your weight onto your left foot. Extend your arms forward and lift your right leg behind you, creating a straight line from your fingertips to your lifted foot. Keep your core engaged and your gaze focused on a point before you. Hold the pose for 20-30 seconds, then switch sides. This pose strengthens your core and legs while enhancing your balance and concentration (Iyengar, 2001).

The Eagle Pose, or Garudasana, challenges your balance and coordination. Stand with your feet together and bend your knees slightly. If possible, lift your right foot and cross it over your left thigh, hooking your right foot behind your left calf. Bring your arms in front of you and cross your right arm under your left, bringing your palms together. Focus on a point in front of you and hold the pose for 20-30 seconds, then switch sides. This pose improves your balance, stretches your shoulders and hips, and enhances your focus (Harvard Health Publishing, 2021).

Half-Moon Pose, or Ardha Chandrasana, is a dynamic pose that improves balance and flexibility. Stand with your feet together and step your right foot back into a lunge. Place your left hand on the floor or on a block about a foot in front of your left foot. Shift your weight onto your left foot and lift your right leg parallel to the floor. Extend your right arm towards the ceiling and turn your gaze upward if comfortable. Hold the pose for 20-30 seconds, then switch sides. This pose strengthens your legs, improves balance, and opens your chest and hips (Iyengar, 2001).

Practicing yoga safely is essential to avoid injury and get the most out of your practice. Using props like blocks and straps can provide additional support and make poses more accessible. For example, placing a block under your hand in Half-Moon Pose can help you maintain balance. Practicing near a wall for support is also helpful, especially when trying new poses. The wall can provide stability and confidence, allowing you to focus on the pose without worrying about falling (Mayo Clinic, 2020).

Focusing on gradual progress is crucial. Yoga is not about pushing yourself to the limit but finding a balance that feels right for you. Start with comfortable poses and gradually work up to more challenging ones. Listening to your body and avoiding overexertion is critical. If a pose feels painful or uncomfortable, modify it or skip it altogether. The goal is to create a practice that supports your well-being and helps you feel good in your body.

Yoga offers a holistic approach to improving balance and overall well-being. With its focus on postures, breath control, and meditation, yoga enhances body awareness, strengthens core muscles, increases flexibility, and reduces stress. You can improve your stability and confidence by practicing balance-focused poses like Tree Pose, Warrior III, Eagle Pose, and Half-Moon Pose. Remember to use props, practice near a wall, focus on gradual progress, and listen to your body to ensure a safe and effective yoga practice.

### 6.5 Safety Tips for Balance Exercises

Safety in balance exercises is not just a good practice; it is a necessity. When you prioritize safety, you prevent falls and injuries, which are crucial for maintaining your independence and overall well-being. Ensuring a safe exercise environment allows you to focus on the movements and build confidence in your abilities. This confidence is essential as it encourages you to keep practicing and improving. Feeling secure in your environment makes the exercises more enjoyable and less stressful, fostering a positive attitude towards physical activity (American College of Sports Medicine, 2021).

Creating a safe exercise space starts with removing any tripping hazards. Look around the area where you plan to exercise and clear away loose rugs, electrical cords, and any clutter that could cause you to trip. Ensuring adequate lighting is also vital. A well-lit space helps you see clearly, reducing the risk of missteps and falls. If you exercise in the evening or early morning, make sure to turn on lights or use additional lighting. Using non-slip mats can provide extra stability, especially if you are exercising on a hard surface like tile or wood. These mats help prevent slips and offer a comfortable surface for your feet. Having a stable chair or support nearby is another excellent precaution, as it allows you to grab onto something if you feel unsteady, giving you the confidence to try new exercises without fear (Harvard Health Publishing, 2021).

Wearing supportive and comfortable shoes can make a big difference. Look for shoes with good arch support and cushioning to absorb shock. Avoid shoes with slippery soles, as they can increase the risk of slipping. Instead, choose shoes with a broad base and a non-slip sole for better stability. Your footwear should fit well and provide ample support to your feet to improve your balance and reduce the strain on your feet and joints during exercises (Mayo Clinic, 2020).

When starting balance exercises, it's essential to begin with simple movements and gradually increase the difficulty. This approach helps your body adapt and build strength without overwhelming it. Staying hydrated is another critical aspect. Drinking enough water before, during, and after exercise keeps your muscles and joints lubricated and functioning well. Dehydration can lead to dizziness and fatigue, increasing the risk of falls. Listening to your body and resting when needed is crucial. Pay attention to how you feel during exercises. If you experience pain or discomfort, stop and rest. Pushing through pain can lead to injuries, so taking breaks and adjusting your routine as needed is better. Consulting a healthcare provider before starting a new exercise routine is necessary for anyone with existing medical issues. They can provide personalized advice based on your health condition and ensure that the exercises you plan to do are safe for you (Harvard Health Publishing, 2021).

7

# Strength Training: Building Muscle Safely

At age 67, Jane noticed a decline in her leg strength that alarmed her. The tasks that once felt effortless, like ascending stairs and carrying groceries, had become daunting challenges. This realization ignited a determination within her to reclaim the robustness of her younger years. In her quest for solutions, Jane discovered the power of strength training. She learned that using multiple methods can promote strength training and provide muscle growth at any age. We will begin this section by exploring how to use body weight through exercises to enhance muscle mass without requiring specialized equipment.

### 7.1 Bodyweight Exercises for Strength

Bodyweight exercises are a fantastic option, especially for seniors. One of the most significant advantages is that no equipment is needed. You can do these exercises anywhere, whether at home, in the park, or even traveling. This convenience makes it easier to stick to a routine. Another significant benefit is the low risk of injury. Since you're using your own body as resistance, it's easier to maintain control and avoid overexertion. These exercises are also highly practical for building functional strength, which helps with everyday activities like lifting, bending, and walking (Harvard Health Publishing, 2019).

Let's dive into some essential bodyweight exercises that are particularly suitable for seniors. Squats are a great place to start. They target your legs and glutes, which are crucial for mobility and balance. To perform a squat:

1. Stand with your feet shoulder-width apart.
2. Lower your body as if sitting back into a chair, keeping your knees behind your toes.
3. Push through your heels to return to the starting position.
4. Aim for 10-15 repetitions to begin with.

Push-ups are another excellent exercise. If the traditional push-up is too challenging, try a wall push-up. Stand a few feet away from a wall, place your hands on the wall at shoulder height, and lean in. Lower your body towards the wall by bending your elbows, then push back to the starting position. This exercise targets your chest, shoulders, and triceps. Start with 8-12 repetitions (American College of Sports Medicine [ACSM], 2021).

Lunges are effective for building leg strength and improving balance. Stand with your feet together, then step forward with one leg and lower your body until both knees are bent at about 90 degrees. Push back to the starting position and switch legs. Ensure your front knee doesn't extend past your toes to avoid strain. Start with 8-10 repetitions on each leg (Mayo Clinic, 2021).

Pull-ups might seem intimidating, but modified versions can make them accessible. For an inverted row, you can use a sturdy table or a low bar. Lie underneath, grasp the edge or bar, and pull your chest towards it. This exercise strengthens your back and arms. Aim for 6-10 repetitions to start (Harvard Health Publishing, 2019).

Planks are fantastic for core strength. Lie face down, then lift your body onto your toes and forearms, keeping your body in a straight line. Hold this position while engaging your core. Start with 20-30 seconds and gradually increase the duration as you get stronger (ACSM, 2021).

Maintaining proper form is crucial to getting the most out of these exercises. Keep your chest up for squats, and avoid letting your knees collapse inward. With push-ups, ensure your body remains in a straight line from head to heels. For lunges, keep your torso upright and your knees aligned with your toes. When performing pull-ups or inverted rows, focus on squeezing your shoulder blades together. During planks, engage your core and avoid letting your hips sag (Mayo Clinic, 2021).

Progressing in bodyweight exercises is all about gradually increasing the challenge. Start by increasing the number of repetitions. If you begin with 10 squats, aim to add one or two more each week. Another way to progress is by adding variations. For example, single-leg squats can add intensity. You can also reduce rest time between sets to keep your muscles engaged. Once you're comfortable with wall push-ups, try moving to knee push-ups and eventually to full push-ups (Harvard Health Publishing, 2019).

For a more interactive approach, consider keeping a workout journal. Note down the exercises you perform, the number of repetitions, and any observations about how you feel so you can track your progress and stay motivated. Remember, consistency is key. Even minor, incremental improvements can lead to significant gains in strength and overall fitness (ACSM, 2021).

Here is your text with appropriate APA citations and a reference list:

### 7.2 Using Resistance Bands: An Affordable Option

Imagine having a compact, versatile tool that can provide a full-body workout without taking up much space in your home. That's precisely what resistance bands offer. These stretchy elastic bands are not only affordable but also incredibly portable. When you complete your routine, you can tuck them into a drawer or even take them on vacation. Their affordability makes them accessible to everyone, and their portability means you can keep up with your fitness routine no matter where you are.

The versatility of resistance bands is another major advantage. Exercise bands are used for a wide range of exercises targeting various muscle groups. Whether you're looking to strengthen your arms, legs, or core, there's an exercise for that. Plus, resistance bands come in different levels of resistance, so you can easily adjust the difficulty of your workouts. If you need more of a challenge, simply use a band with higher resistance. This adjustability is particularly beneficial for seniors, as it allows you to start slow and gradually increase the intensity as you build strength. Importantly, resistance bands are low impact, which means they put less strain on your joints than weights, making them a safer option for many older adults (Harvard Health Publishing, 2019).

Let's look at some critical resistance band exercises that you can incorporate into your routine. Bicep curls are a great way to strengthen your arms. Stand on the middle of the band and hold the handles with your palms facing up. Keeping your elbows close to your sides, curl your hands towards your shoulders. This movement targets your biceps and can help improve your ability to lift and carry objects in daily life.

Seated rows are excellent for your back and shoulders. Sit on the floor with extended legs and loop the band around your feet. Pull the handles towards your torso, squeezing your shoulder blades together. This exercise strengthens your upper back and improves posture, which is crucial for preventing back pain and maintaining balance (American College of Sports Medicine [ACSM], 2021).

Lateral band walks are perfect for targeting your hip muscles and improving stability. Place the band around your legs just above your knees. Stand with your feet shoulder-width apart and then take small steps to the side, keeping tension on the band. This exercise helps strengthen the muscles around your hips, improving your balance and reducing the risk of falls.

Chest presses can be done either standing or lying down. Anchor the band behind you and hold the handles at chest level with your elbows bent. Press the handles forward until your arms are fully extended, then return to the starting position. This exercise targets your chest and triceps, helping you build upper body strength (Harvard Health Publishing, 2019).

It's essential to secure resistance bands properly so they can be used safely and effectively. Make sure it's anchored firmly to avoid slipping. When performing exercises, maintain control at all times. Avoid letting the band snap back quickly, as this can cause injury. Adjust the band tension to match your fitness level. Switch to a band with higher resistance if an exercise feels too easy. Proper breathing techniques are also important. Exhale during the exertion phase of the exercise, such as when you're lifting or pressing, and inhale during the relaxation phase (Mayo Clinic, 2021).

Incorporating resistance bands into your regular workout routine can be incredibly effective. Incorporate these exercises into your weekly regimen and maintain a workout journal to monitor your strength and endurance enhancements. Given their cost-effectiveness, ease of storage, and adaptability, resistance bands are an excellent choice for any fitness plan, particularly for seniors aiming to increase strength in a safe manner.

### 7.3 Light Weight Training: Building Muscle Gradually

Light weight training offers an excellent way to build muscle without overloading your joints. Weight training is particularly beneficial for seniors, as it reduces the risk of injury while providing the resistance needed to strengthen muscles. Using light weights can also improve bone density, an essential factor in preventing osteoporosis. Regular training will enhance muscle endurance, making everyday activities like carrying groceries or climbing stairs easier. Light weight exercises are versatile, allowing you to focus on different muscle groups and adjust the intensity as you progress (Harvard Health Publishing, 2021).

One of the important exercises in light weight training is the dumbbell shoulder press. This exercise targets your shoulders and arms. Start by selecting an appropriate weight for beginners, typically between 2 to 5 pounds. Stand with your feet shoulder-width apart, holding a dumbbell in each hand. Raise the dumbbells to shoulder height, palms facing forward. Press the weights upward until your arms are fully extended, then lower them back to the starting position. Keep your core engaged, and avoid arching your back. Aim for 8-12 repetitions to begin with (American College of Sports Medicine [ACSM], 2021).

Tricep extensions are another excellent exercise for building arm strength. To perform this exercise:

1. Sit on a chair with a dumbbell in one hand.
2. Raise the dumbbell above your head, then bend your elbow to lower the weight behind your head.
3. Extend your arm back to the starting position.

This movement targets the triceps, the muscles on the back of your upper arm. Ensure you keep your elbow close to your head and avoid flaring it out. Start with 8-12 repetitions for each arm (Mayo Clinic, 2021).

Weighted leg raises focus on strengthening your legs and core. Lie on your back with extended legs and a light weight secured between your feet. Slowly lift your legs towards the ceiling, keeping them straight. Lower them back down without letting them touch the floor. This exercise targets the lower abdominal muscles and hip flexors. Keep your movements controlled, and avoid using momentum. Aim for 10-15 repetitions (Harvard Health Publishing, 2021).

Bent-over rows are great for your back and shoulders. Stand with your feet shoulder-width apart, holding a dumbbell in each hand. Bend your knees slightly and hinge forward at the hips, keeping your back straight. Let the dumbbells hang down in front of you. Pull the weights towards your torso, squeezing your shoulder blades together, then lower them back down. This exercise helps improve posture and strengthen the upper back. Start with 8-12 repetitions (ACSM, 2021).

When selecting an appropriate weight, consider starting light and gradually increasing as you become more comfortable with the movements. For beginners, 2 to 5 pounds is usually a good starting point. Ensure you can perform the exercises with proper form before increasing the weight. Each exercise has a specific starting position, so take the time to set yourself up correctly. For example, when performing the dumbbell shoulder press, ensure your feet are shoulder-width apart, and your core is engaged.

Maintaining proper form is crucial to prevent injury and maximize the effectiveness of each exercise. For the shoulder press, keep your wrists straight and avoid locking your elbows at the top of the movement. Keep your elbow close to your head during tricep extensions and avoid arching your back. In weighted leg raises, ensure your lower back stays pressed into the floor to engage your core properly. For bent-over rows, keep your back straight and avoid rounding your shoulders (Mayo Clinic, 2021).

Progression in light weight training involves gradually increasing the weight and intensity of your exercises. Start by adding more sets and repetitions. If you begin with one set of 8-12 repetitions, aim to increase to two or three sets over time. Once you're comfortable with the current weight, try increasing it by 1-2 pounds. Incorporating compound movements can also add intensity. For example, combine a dumbbell shoulder press with a squat to engage multiple muscle groups simultaneously, making the workout more challenging and efficient.

By following these steps and maintaining consistency, you'll see significant improvements in your strength and overall fitness. Light weight training offers a safe and effective way to build muscle, improve bone density, and enhance muscle endurance, making it an ideal option for seniors looking to stay active and healthy.

### 7.4 Blood Flow Restriction Training: A New Approach to Weight Training

Blood Flow Restriction (BFR) training is a fascinating method that has gained traction recently, especially among older adults. The concept is straightforward: you use bands to partially restrict blood flow to the muscles you're working; while this might sound counterintuitive, it actually enhances muscle growth with lighter weights. Because the blood flow is restricted, your muscles experience stress similar to lifting heavier weights, making BFR training particularly appealing for those who find traditional weightlifting challenging. You can achieve significant muscle gains with much lighter weights, reducing the risk of injury (Hughes et al., 2017).

One of the standout benefits of BFR training is that it reduces the risk of joint strain. For seniors, joint health is paramount, and heavy lifting can sometimes exacerbate joint issues. With BFR, you can get the benefits of heavy lifting without the associated risks. The technique also accelerates muscle hypertrophy or muscle growth. This is because the restricted blood flow causes a buildup of metabolites that promote muscle growth (Loenneke et al., 2016).

Additionally, BFR training improves recovery times. The lighter weights mean less overall stress on your body, allowing for quicker recovery between sessions and making it easier to maintain a consistent workout routine (Slysz et al., 2016).

To safely perform BFR training, it's crucial to position the bands correctly. Place the bands at the top of the limb you're working on —just below the shoulder for arms and below the hip for legs. The goal is to restrict blood flow without cutting it off entirely. You should still be able to feel a pulse below the band. Choosing appropriate exercises is also essential. Bicep curls, leg extensions, and tricep pushdowns are excellent choices because they isolate the muscles effectively. Monitoring pressure levels is vital. The bands should be tight enough to restrict blood flow but not so tight that they cause numbness or pain. Start with moderate pressure and adjust as needed (Hughes et al., 2017).

Regarding duration and frequency, keep your BFR sessions short but frequent. Aim for 15-20 minutes per session, two to three times a week. This allows you to reap the benefits without overdoing it. Always listen to your body and give yourself time to recover between sessions. A good rule of thumb is to wait 48 hours before working the same muscle group again. Proper recovery ensures that your muscles have enough time to recover and grow (Loenneke et al., 2016).

Here's a sample BFR workout routine to get you started. Begin with bicep curls using light weights. Stand with your feet shoulder-width apart and hold a dumbbell in each hand. Place the BFR bands just below your shoulders and perform the curls, aiming for 15-20 repetitions. Next, move on to leg extensions. Sit on a chair or bench with the bands placed just below your hips. Extend one leg at a time, focusing on squeezing the muscles at the top of the movement. Aim for 15-20 repetitions on each leg.

Tricep pushdowns are another excellent exercise to include. Use a resistance band or cable machine and place the BFR bands below your shoulders. Push the band or cable down until your arms are fully extended, then return to the starting position. Aim for 15-20 repetitions. Throughout your workout, continually monitor and adjust the band tightness. They should be snug but not painfully tight. If you experience any numbness or tingling, loosen the bands immediately.

Remember, the goal is to create a safe and effective workout environment. Start with lighter weights and shorter sessions, gradually increasing as you become more comfortable with the technique. By incorporating BFR training into your routine, you can achieve significant muscle growth and improved strength with less risk of injury, making it an excellent option for seniors.

## 7.5 Strength Training Safety and Modifications

When you start strength training, safety should be your top priority. This is especially true for seniors, as the risks of injury can be higher. Preventing injury is crucial, not just for your immediate well-being but also to ensure that you can continue exercising long-term. An injury can set you back weeks or even months, so taking precautions is essential. Ensuring long-term adherence to your exercise routine is another reason why safety matters. You're more likely to stick with your workouts when you feel safe and confident. Building confidence in your abilities can transform your exercise experience into something you look forward to rather than dread (American College of Sports Medicine [ACSM], 2021).

To practice strength training safely, start with a proper warm-up which gets your blood flowing and prepares your muscles for the work ahead. Simple activities like marching in place or gentle arm circles can be effective. Using proper form is another critical aspect. Incorrect form can lead to strains or other injuries. If you need more clarification about your form, consider working with a trainer, even if it's just for a few sessions. Listening to your body is equally important. Pain is your body's way of telling you something is wrong. If you feel sharp or persistent pain, stop the exercise and consult a healthcare provider. Staying hydrated is also crucial. Dehydration can lead to dizziness or muscle cramps, increasing the risk of injury (Harvard Health Publishing, 2019).

Strength training exercises can be adapted to suit different fitness levels and health conditions. For example, if you find traditional squats challenging, use a chair for support. Stand behind the chair and hold onto the backrest while you perform the squats to help you maintain balance and reduce the risk of falling. Reducing the range of motion is another way to modify exercises. If lunges are too difficult, try a half-lunge instead. Lower yourself only partway down, gradually increasing the depth as you become stronger. Using lighter weights or less resistance is also a viable modification. If you're using resistance bands or light weights, start with the lowest resistance and increase it gradually. Finally, consider increasing rest periods between sets to give your muscles time to recover and reduce the risk of overexertion (ACSM, 2021).

Monitoring your progress is vital for making adjustments and staying motivated. Keeping a workout journal can be incredibly helpful. Note down the exercises you perform, the number of sets and repetitions, and how you feel afterward. This journal can help you track improvements and identify areas that need more focus. Regularly reassessing your fitness levels is also essential. Every few weeks, take a moment to evaluate your progress. Are you lifting heavier weights? Can you do more repetitions? These indicators can help you adjust your routine to keep it challenging. Celebrating small milestones is essential for maintaining motivation. Did you manage to add an extra set of push-ups? Celebrate it! Small victories add up and keep you moving forward (Harvard Health Publishing, 2019).

As you incorporate these safety tips and modifications into your strength training routine, remember that consistency is required. Small, steady progress is better than pushing yourself too hard and risking injury. The goal is to build strength safely and sustainably, ensuring you enjoy an active, fulfilling life. With the proper precautions and a mindful approach, strength training can be a powerful tool for improving your overall health and well-being (Harvard Health Publishing, 2019).

Embarking on a strength training regimen is akin to setting out on a transformative journey—one that demands patience, unwavering dedication, and an unwavering commitment to safety. By placing these principles at the forefront of your fitness endeavors, you are effectively laying a solid foundation for enduring success. This approach ensures a safer experience and cultivates a sense of achievement and progress as you advance (American College of Sports Medicine [ACSM], 2021).

In the forthcoming chapter, we will explore a wide range of advanced exercise techniques. These will infuse your workout routine with exciting variety and challenge your body in new ways, ensuring that your path to physical well-being remains engaging and rewarding.

# 8

# Advanced Exercise Techniques: Keeping It Interesting

Imagine standing in your living room, the upbeat music playing, and moving your feet to a rhythm you haven't felt in years. That's the power of aerobic exercise. For many seniors, getting the heart pumping might seem daunting, but it's one of the most beneficial forms of exercise you can incorporate into your routine. Aerobic exercise is crucial for cardiovascular health and overall well-being. It improves heart health by strengthening the heart muscle and enhancing its ability to pump blood efficiently. Getting your heart pumping means better circulation and lower blood pressure, reducing the risk of heart disease. Additionally, aerobic exercise enhances lung capacity, making everyday activities like climbing stairs or carrying groceries easier. You'll find yourself breathing more deeply and easily, which can be incredibly invigorating (American Heart Association, 2018).

Moreover, engaging in regular aerobic exercise boosts energy levels. You might think that expending energy in exercise would leave you feeling tired, but it's quite the opposite. Aerobic activities increase the production of endorphins, the body's natural mood enhancers, which can leave you feeling more energized and positive. This boost in energy can translate to better productivity and enjoyment in your daily activities (Harvard Health Publishing, 2019). Additionally, aerobic exercise aids in weight management. As you get your heart rate up and keep it elevated, you burn calories, which helps shed those extra pounds. Maintaining a healthy weight reduces the risk of many chronic diseases, including diabetes and hypertension, making you feel lighter and more agile (Mayo Clinic, 2021).

There are various types of aerobic exercises that you can try. Low-impact aerobics are perfect if you're concerned about joint health. These exercises are gentle on the joints but effective in increasing your heart rate. Dance-based workouts are another fun option. Whether it's Zumba or a simple dance routine, moving to music can make exercise feel less like a chore and more like a party. Step aerobics involves using a raised platform to step up and down, which can be an excellent workout for the legs and cardiovascular system. Circuit training combines different aerobic exercises in a sequence, giving you a full-body workout. Each option provides a unique way to keep your routine interesting and engaging (American College of Sports Medicine [ACSM], 2021).

Let's walk through a basic aerobics routine. Start with a warm-up by marching in place for about five minutes to get your blood flowing and prepare your muscles for the workout. Once you're warmed up, move into the main workout. Begin with step touches: step one foot to the side, bring the other foot to meet it, and repeat on the other side. Next, try side steps: step one foot to the side while bringing your arms up and down, then step the other foot to meet it.

Finally, add grapevines:

- Step one foot to the side.
- Cross the other foot behind.
- Step out again with the first foot.
- Bring the other foot to meet it.

These moves are simple yet effective in raising your heart rate. End your session with a cool-down, doing gentle stretching to relax your muscles and gradually lower your heart rate (Harvard Health Publishing, 2019).

As you progress in your aerobic exercise, gradually increasing the intensity and duration is important. Start by extending your session length by a few minutes each week to help build stamina without overwhelming your body. Adding more complex moves can also increase intensity. For example, you can incorporate light hand weights during step touches and side steps to engage your upper body more. Joining group aerobics classes can be a fantastic way to stay motivated and make exercise a social activity. Many community centers and gyms offer classes specifically designed for seniors, ensuring the exercises are appropriate and safe for your fitness level (Mayo Clinic, 2021).

### 8.1 Interactive Element: Personal Aerobics Progress Tracker

Use this tracker to monitor your progress and stay motivated. Fill in your goals and achievements weekly.

**Week 1 Goals:**

- Warm-up: March in place for 5 minutes
- Main workout: Step-touches, side steps, grapevines (15 minutes total)

- Cool-down: Gentle stretching (5 minutes)

**Achievements:**

- Monday:
- Tuesday:
- Wednesday:
- Thursday:
- Friday:
- Saturday:
- Sunday:

**Week 2 Goals:**

- Warm-up: March in place for 5 minutes
- Main workout: Step-touches, side steps, grapevines (20 minutes total)
- Cool-down: Gentle stretching (5 minutes)

**Achievements:**

- Monday:
- Tuesday:
- Wednesday:
- Thursday:
- Friday:
- Saturday:
- Sunday:

Keep this tracker handy to see how far you've come and to encourage yourself to keep going. Each step forward is a victory, no matter how small.

## 8.2 Elliptical and Treadmill Workouts

Imagine stepping onto an elliptical or treadmill, knowing these tools can transform your fitness journey. For seniors, these machines offer numerous benefits. One of the most significant advantages is that they are low-impact on your joints. Unlike running on hard pavement, which can be hard on your knees and hips, ellipticals and treadmills provide a cushioned surface that absorbs shock and makes them ideal for those with arthritis or joint pain. Additionally, both machines come with adjustable intensity levels. Whether you're just starting or looking to push your limits, you can customize the resistance and speed to match your fitness level (American College of Sports Medicine [ACSM], 2021). They also provide an indoor exercise option, which is perfect for days when the weather isn't cooperating. You can stay consistent with your workouts without worrying about rain, snow, or extreme heat. Another significant benefit is the built-in workout programs that many of these machines offer. These programs can guide you through various workouts, keeping your routine fresh and challenging.

Using an elliptical effectively involves a few key tips. First, adjust the resistance and incline to match your fitness level. If you're new to using an elliptical, start with a lower resistance and gradually increase it as you build strength and endurance. Maintaining proper posture is crucial. Stand up straight, engage your core, and avoid leaning too heavily on the handlebars to ensure you're working the right muscle groups and reducing the risk of injury (Harvard Health Publishing, 2020). Speaking of handlebars, remember to use them for upper-body engagement. Pushing and pulling the handlebars can work your arms, shoulders, and chest, making your workout more comprehensive. Monitoring your heart rate is also important. Most ellipticals come with built-in heart rate monitors. Aim to stay within your target heart rate zone to maximize cardiovascular benefits and ensure you're working at an appropriate intensity.

Treadmills offer a variety of workout options to keep things interesting. A straightforward way to use a treadmill is to walk at different speeds. Start slowly, comfortably warm up, then gradually increase your speed to challenge your cardiovascular system. Incline walking is another effective method to add intensity. Raising the incline mimics uphill walking, which engages your leg muscles more and burns more calories (Mayo Clinic, 2021). Interval training is a great way to boost your fitness. Alternate between periods of high-intensity walking or light jogging and slower recovery periods. Using a treadmill this way keeps your workout engaging, improves your cardiovascular health, and burns more calories in less time. You can incorporate light jogging into your treadmill routine if you're comfortable. Start with short jogging intervals and gradually increase the duration as your fitness improves.

Here's a sample workout plan that combines both elliptical and treadmill exercises. Begin with a warm-up of five minutes of slow walking, which helps get your blood flowing and prepares your muscles for the workout. For the main workout, spend 20 minutes alternating between walking and incline walking on the treadmill. Start with two minutes of walking at a comfortable pace, then switch to two minutes of walking on a higher incline. Repeat this cycle for 20 minutes. If you're using an elliptical, you can follow a similar pattern by alternating between low and high resistance. Finally, finish with five minutes of slow walking and stretching cool-down to help your body recover and reduce muscle stiffness.

This structured plan provides a balanced approach to cardio, ensuring you get the benefits of both machines. The variety also keeps the routine interesting, making sticking with your fitness goals easier.

### 8.3 Vibration Plate: Enhancing Exercise Benefits

Imagine stepping onto a platform that gently vibrates beneath your feet. This is a vibration plate, a piece of equipment that vibrates at various frequencies to enhance your workouts. These vibrations cause your muscles to contract rapidly, providing a workout that can be more effective in less time. Another great benefit of a vibration plate is the engagement of the lymph system. After years of a sedentary lifestyle, our lymph system often gets stagnant and doesn't work to remove waste from our system as designed. Vibration plates send energy waves through your body, forcing your muscles to contract and relax multiple times per second, enhancing muscle contraction and improving circulation, bringing more oxygen and nutrients to your tissues (Harvard Health Publishing, 2020). Additionally, the vibrations help accelerate recovery by reducing muscle soreness and stiffness.

For seniors, the benefits of using a vibration plate are numerous. One of the most notable advantages is increased muscle strength. Rapid muscle contractions stimulated by vibrations help build and tone muscles, even with minimal movement. This can be particularly beneficial if you have mobility issues or find traditional strength training exercises challenging. Improved balance and coordination are other significant benefits. The instability created by the vibrations forces your body to engage stabilizer muscles, which enhances your balance and coordination over time and can be especially important in preventing falls and maintaining independence (Mayo Clinic, 2021).

Another advantage of vibration plate exercises is reduced joint pain. The gentle vibrations can help alleviate joint discomfort by promoting better circulation and reducing inflammation, making them an excellent option for arthritis or other joint-related issues. Enhanced flexibility is also a key benefit. The vibrations help loosen tight muscles and increase range of motion, making it easier to perform daily activities and other forms of exercise.

Let's look at some specific exercises you can do on a vibration plate. Squats are a great starting point. Stand on the plate with your feet shoulder-width apart. Lower your body as if sitting back into a chair, keeping your knees behind your toes. Hold the squat for a few seconds before standing back up. Repeat this movement to strengthen your legs and glutes. Calf raises are another effective exercise. Stand on the plate with your feet shoulder-width apart. Lift your heels off the ground, rising onto your toes, then lower them back down to target your calf muscles and improve your stability.

Plank holds are excellent for engaging your core muscles. Place your forearms on the vibration plate and extend your legs behind you, keeping your body straight from head to heels. Hold this position, ensuring your core is tight and your back is flat. This exercise helps to strengthen your core, improve posture, and support overall stability. Seated leg lifts are another simple yet effective exercise. Sit on the edge of the vibration plate with your feet flat on the ground. Lift one leg at a time, holding it in the air for a few seconds before lowering it back down. This exercise targets your lower abs and hip flexors, helping to improve strength and flexibility.

Safety is paramount when using a vibration plate. Start with low-frequency settings to allow your body to adjust to the vibrations. Keeping sessions short initially, around 5 to 10 minutes, helps your body get used to the new form of exercise without overexertion. Using the vibration plate as part of a balanced routine and incorporating other forms of exercise like walking, strength training, and stretching is crucial. Multiple forms of balance exercises ensure a well-rounded workout that addresses all aspects of fitness. Finally, always consult with your healthcare provider before starting any new exercise program, especially if you have underlying health conditions. They can provide personalized advice and ensure that vibration plate exercises are safe for you (Harvard Health Publishing, 2020).

This advanced technique uniquely enhances your fitness routine, making building strength, improving balance, and reducing joint pain easier. By following these guidelines and incorporating vibration plate exercises into your workouts, you can enjoy a more effective and enjoyable fitness regimen.

### 8.4 Aquatic Exercises: Low-Impact, High-Benefit

Imagine stepping into a pool, the cool water enveloping you, making you feel weightless. For many seniors, this is a refreshing experience and a gateway to a whole new way of exercising. Aquatic exercises are excellent for seniors for several reasons. First, they are low-impact on your joints, making them ideal for arthritis or joint pain. The buoyancy of the water supports your body, reducing the strain on your joints and minimizing the risk of injury, allowing you to move more freely and with less discomfort (American College of Sports Medicine [ACSM], 2021).

Another significant advantage is the natural resistance provided by water. Every movement you make in the water encounters resistance, which helps to strengthen your muscles without the need for weights. Aquatic exercise provides evenly distributed resistance, ensuring a balanced workout for your entire body (Mayo Clinic, 2021). Additionally, the cooling effect of water helps to prevent overheating. Unlike land-based exercises, where you might quickly feel hot and sweaty, the water regulates your body temperature, allowing you to exercise for longer periods.

Enhancing mobility and flexibility is another important benefit of aquatic exercises. The water allows you to move your joints through a full range of motion, which can help improve your flexibility. Flexibility is essential for daily functional movements like bending, reaching, and walking. The supportive environment of the pool makes it easier to perform stretching and flexibility exercises, which can help reduce stiffness and improve overall mobility (Harvard Health Publishing, 2020).

You can try several types of aquatic exercises, each offering unique benefits. Water walking or jogging is a great starting point. Walk or jog in the pool's shallow end, using the water's resistance to strengthen your legs and improve your cardiovascular health. Aqua aerobics classes are another excellent option. These classes typically involve aerobic movements performed in the water, such as jumping jacks and leg lifts. The buoyancy of the water reduces the impact on your joints, making these exercises accessible and enjoyable (American Heart Association, 2018).

Pool yoga combines the principles of yoga with the benefits of water. The water's buoyancy supports your body, allowing you to perform yoga poses with greater ease and stability, which can help improve your balance, flexibility, and strength. Swimming laps is another fantastic way to get a full-body workout. Whether you prefer freestyle, backstroke, or breaststroke, swimming engages multiple muscle groups and provides a great cardiovascular workout.

Let's dive into a simple aquatic exercise routine. Start with a warm-up by gently walking in the water for about five minutes. Walking helps get your blood flowing and prepares your muscles for the workout. The main workout begins with water jogging.

Move your legs as if jogging on land, keeping your upper body upright and using your arms for balance. Next, try leg lifts. Stand in the water, lift one leg to the side, and lower it back down. Repeat on the other side. This exercise strengthens your hip muscles and improves your balance. Finally, add arm circles. Stand in the water with your arms extended out to the sides. Make small circles with your arms, gradually increasing the size of the circles. This helps to strengthen your shoulder muscles and improve your range of motion.

End your session with a cool-down by floating and stretching in the water. Lie on your back and let the water support you. Stretch your arms and legs out, feeling the gentle pull of the water. The water helps relax your muscles and reduce any tension during the workout.

As you become more comfortable with aquatic exercises, you can gradually increase the intensity and variety. Water weights are one way to add resistance and challenge your muscles further. Start with light water weights and incorporate them into your exercises, such as holding them while water jogging or using them during arm circles. Increasing the duration of your sessions is another way to progress. Start with shorter sessions and gradually extend the time as your endurance improves.

Joining a water aerobics class can also be a fun and social way to stay motivated. These classes, taught by trained instructors, can guide you through various exercises and ensure you're performing them correctly. Incorporating swimming drills into your routine can add variety and challenge. Try different strokes or set goals for how many laps you want to complete.

Aquatic exercises offer a low-impact, high-benefit way to stay active and improve your overall health. Whether you're walking in the water, joining an aqua aerobics class, practicing pool yoga, or swimming laps, you'll find that the supportive environment of the pool makes it easier and more enjoyable to stay fit. So, next time you have the opportunity, take a dip in the pool and discover the benefits of aquatic exercises for yourself.

## 8.5 Combining Techniques for a Holistic Routine

Imagine waking up each morning excited about your daily exercise, knowing that today will bring something new and engaging. One of the most effective ways to maintain this enthusiasm is by combining different exercise techniques into a varied routine. This approach prevents boredom, keeping your workouts fresh and exciting. Mixing things up makes you more likely to stick with your exercise plan, making it a sustainable habit rather than a chore (American College of Sports Medicine [ACSM], 2021). But the benefits go beyond just staying interested. A varied exercise routine engages different muscle groups, ensuring a well-rounded fitness experience. You enhance your overall strength, flexibility, and endurance by targeting various parts of your body.

Another significant advantage is that a diverse exercise routine reduces the risk of overuse injuries. When you perform the same exercises repeatedly, you put stress on the same muscles and joints, increasing the likelihood of injury. By incorporating different workout types, you give specific muscle groups time to recover while still staying active. This balance helps protect your body from wear and tear, making maintaining a consistent exercise regimen easier (Harvard Health Publishing, 2019). Moreover, a varied routine enhances overall fitness. Each type of exercise offers unique benefits, from improving cardiovascular health and building muscle strength to increasing flexibility and balance. By combining these techniques, you create a holistic approach that addresses all aspects of fitness.

Creating a balanced exercise plan involves thoughtful scheduling and utilizing various workouts. Start by scheduling different types of exercises on different days. For example, dedicate one day to strength training, another to cardio, and another to flexibility exercises. This variation keeps your routine interesting and ensures you work on different fitness components. Balancing strength, cardio, and flexibility exercises is crucial. Strength training builds muscle and enhances metabolism, cardio improves heart health and endurance, and flexibility exercises increase your range of motion and reduce stiffness. Including all three in your weekly plan provides a comprehensive fitness approach (Mayo Clinic, 2020).

Proper rest and recovery are also essential. Rest days give your muscles time to repair and grow, reducing the risk of injury and preventing burnout. Listen to your body and adjust your plan as needed. If you're feeling particularly sore or tired, take an extra rest day or opt for a gentle stretching session instead of a more intense workout. This flexibility ensures you're not pushing yourself too hard and helps maintain a positive relationship with exercise.

**Sample Weekly Exercise Plan**

- **Monday:** Walking for fitness - Start your week with a brisk walk to increase your heart rate and get the blood flowing. Walking is an excellent way to boost cardiovascular health while being gentle on your joints.
- **Tuesday:** Rest and recovery - Allow your body to rest and recover. Use this day to relax and recharge, ensuring you're ready for the next workout.
- **Wednesday:** Strength training with resistance bands - Focus on building muscle strength using resistance bands.

This type of workout targets multiple muscle groups and helps improve overall strength and stability.
- **Thursday:** Rest and recovery - This is a rest day to give your muscles time to repair. Consider incorporating light stretching or yoga to stay active without overexerting yourself.
- **Friday:** Aquatic exercises - Head to the pool for a low-impact, high-benefit workout. Aquatic exercises are excellent for improving mobility and flexibility while being easy on your joints.
- **Saturday:** Stretching - Dedicate this day to flexibility exercises. Stretching helps reduce muscle tension, improve range of motion, and prevent stiffness.
- **Sunday:** Rest and recovery - Finish the week with a day of rest. Use this time to reflect on your progress and plan for the upcoming week.

Setting short-term and long-term goals keeps you focused and motivated. Short-term goals provide immediate satisfaction, like completing a week of workouts without skipping any days. Long-term goals, like improving your flexibility or increasing your strength, give you something to strive for and can be incredibly rewarding when achieved (Locke & Latham, 2002).

Celebrating milestones is another excellent way to stay motivated. Whether you reach a new personal best in a particular exercise or stick to your plan for a month, take the time to acknowledge and celebrate your achievements. This positive reinforcement encourages you to keep going. Finding an exercise buddy or joining a group can also provide motivation and support. Having someone to share your progress with and hold you accountable makes the experience more enjoyable and less isolating (Harvard Health Publishing, 2019).

Combining different exercise techniques into a holistic routine offers numerous benefits, from keeping your workouts interesting to enhancing overall fitness. By scheduling various workouts, balancing different fitness components, and allowing for proper rest and recovery, you create a sustainable and effective exercise plan. Tracking your progress, setting goals, celebrating milestones, and finding support are all crucial for staying motivated and committed to your fitness journey.

# 9

# Holistic Health: Connecting Mind and Body

Alan, a man who had always cherished his morning coffee and newspaper, became increasingly isolated and doubted his worth as he aged. At his daughter's suggestion, he reluctantly joined her for a walk in the local park. This seemingly simple act of physical activity turned out to be a pivotal moment. Alan realized that exercise wasn't just about moving muscles—it was a potent tool for lifting his spirits and enhancing his mental well-being.

## 9.1 The Mental Benefits of Regular Exercise

Celebrate exercise for its physical benefits, and its impact on mental health is equally profound. When you engage in physical activity, your body releases endorphins, often called "feel-good" hormones. These natural chemicals act as painkillers and mood enhancers, creating a sense of euphoria and reducing feelings of stress. This is why you might hear of a "runner's high" or feel an immediate lift in your mood after a brisk walk (Harvard Health Publishing, 2020).

In addition to endorphin release, regular exercise significantly reduces symptoms of anxiety and depression. Physical activity regulates cortisol and adrenaline stress hormones, promoting a calmer, more balanced emotional state. A study published in the *American Journal of Geriatric Psychiatry* found that seniors who engaged in regular exercise experienced a notable reduction in depressive symptoms (Mather et al., 2002). The researchers noted that even moderate-intensity exercise, such as walking or light aerobics, improved mood and overall mental health.

Exercise also plays a crucial role in maintaining and enhancing cognitive function. Cognitive decline can become a concern as we age, affecting memory, attention, and problem-solving abilities. Physical activity increases blood flow to the brain, promoting neurogenesis, which is the growth of new brain cells. In simpler terms, this means that exercise helps your brain create new cells, which in turn helps improve cognitive function and keeps your mind sharp. According to research, seniors who exercise regularly perform better on cognitive tests and have a lower risk of developing conditions like dementia (National Institute on Aging, 2020).

Moreover, regular exercise can significantly enhance your mood. Physical activity can stimulate the production of neurotransmitters like serotonin and dopamine, which are crucial for mood regulation. Engaging in activities you enjoy, whether dancing, swimming, or gardening, can lead to a happier, more positive outlook on life. You will smile more often, feel more optimistic, and experience greater well-being (Harvard Health Publishing, 2020).

For seniors, the mental health benefits of exercise extend beyond mood improvement. Regular physical activity can decrease feelings of loneliness and isolation. Participating in group exercises,

## Holistic Health: Connecting Mind and Body

walking clubs, or fitness classes creates social interaction and connection opportunities. This sense of community can combat loneliness, providing emotional support and fostering new friendships (Centers for Disease Control and Prevention [CDC], 2021). Additionally, exercise can enhance self-esteem and confidence. Achieving fitness goals, no matter how small, boosts your self-worth and reinforces your ability to make positive changes in your life.

Better sleep quality is another significant benefit of regular exercise. Physical activity helps regulate your sleep-wake cycle, making it easier to fall and stay asleep. Improved sleep quality directly impacts mental health, reducing irritability and enhancing daytime alertness. Seniors who exercise regularly often report feeling more rested and rejuvenated, ready to take on the day's activities (National Sleep Foundation, 2020).

Incorporating exercise into your daily life doesn't have to be daunting. Start by setting specific times for physical activity, making it a non-negotiable part of your routine. Choose activities you enjoy, whether it's taking a morning walk, joining a dance class, or practicing gentle yoga. Begin with small, attainable goals, such as walking for 10 minutes daily and gradually increasing the duration. Use social support to stay motivated—invite friends or family members to join you, or participate in group fitness classes. This sense of community well-being can combat loneliness, provide emotional support, foster new friendships, and make exercise an enjoyable and rewarding part of your daily life.

**Interactive Element: Journaling Prompt**

Keep a daily exercise journal. Note how you feel before and after each activity. Track the types of exercises, duration, and any changes in your mood, energy levels, and sleep quality. Reflect on these entries to identify patterns and celebrate your progress. Remember, every step you take towards better mental health is a reason to celebrate and a sign of your strength and resilience. Tracking your progress is not just about celebrating your achievements; it's also a powerful tool for motivation and adjusting your health routines, putting you in control of your health and well-being (APA, 2017).

Exercising regularly is a powerful tool for enhancing mental health. Exercise releases endorphins, reduces anxiety and depression, improves cognitive function, and promotes better sleep (Harvard Health Publishing, 2020). By incorporating enjoyable activities and leveraging social support, you can experience the profound mental health benefits of regular physical activity.

### 9.2 Stress Reduction Techniques for Seniors

Stress management is crucial as its impact extends beyond feeling overwhelmed. Chronic stress hurts both your physical and mental health, contributing to high blood pressure, weakened immune function, and even heart disease. Mentally, stress can exacerbate anxiety and depression, creating a vicious cycle that affects your overall quality of life (American Psychological Association [APA], 2018). Effective stress management leads to better mental well-being, improved physical health, and a more fulfilling daily experience.

Several effective techniques exist to help manage stress. Deep breathing exercises are a simple yet powerful method. By focusing on your breath, you can calm your mind and body. To practice, sit comfortably, inhale deeply through your nose, hold for a few seconds, and then exhale slowly through your mouth. This technique helps slow your heart rate and relax your muscles, making it an excellent tool for immediate stress relief (National Institute of Mental Health, 2021).

Progressive muscle relaxation is another effective method that involves tensing and relaxing different muscle groups, starting from your toes and working your way up to your head. Find a quiet place to sit or lie down. Begin by tensing the muscles in your feet, hold for a few seconds, then release. Move on to your calves, thighs, and so on until you've covered your entire body. This technique reduces physical tension and promotes a sense of mental calm (Jacobson, 1938).

Mindfulness meditation focuses on being present in the moment. It involves paying attention to your thoughts and feelings without judgment. Find a quiet space, sit comfortably, and close your eyes. Focus on your breath or a simple mantra, like "peace." If your mind wanders, gently bring your focus back. Regular practice can enhance emotional regulation and reduce stress (Kabat-Zinn, 1994).

Guided imagery involves visualizing peaceful and calming scenes. Close your eyes and imagine a serene beach, a lush forest, or any relaxing place. Engage all your senses—imagine the sound of waves, the smell of pine, the feel of a gentle breeze. This technique can transport you away from stress and into a state of relaxation (Naparstek, 1994).

Integrating these techniques into your daily routine can make a significant difference. Set aside dedicated time each day for stress reduction, even if it's just 10 minutes. Use apps or online resources for guided sessions to walk you through these techniques. Combining these practices with soothing activities, like taking a warm bath or walking in nature, can enhance their effectiveness. The key is becoming consistent. Make each of these techniques a regular part of your day; over time, you'll likely notice a reduction in your stress levels, leading to a healthier, happier life.

## 9.3 Mind-Body Exercises: Meditation

Mind-body exercises like meditation offer a unique blend of physical and mental benefits, creating a harmonious connection between the mind and body. Mind-body exercises promote physical and psychological harmony by encouraging you to focus on the present moment, enhancing self-awareness, and reducing stress and anxiety (Kabat-Zinn, 1994). When you meditate, you create a space to tune into your body and mind, noticing how they interact and influence one another. This heightened awareness can lead to improved focus and concentration as you learn to quiet the mental chatter and be fully present.

Mental clarity is another key benefit of meditation. Focusing on your breathing helps to clear the mind, making it easier to concentrate and think clearly (Harvard Health Publishing, 2020).

Meditation provides additional mental benefits. Focused attention meditation is a simple technique that concentrates on a single focus point, such as your breath, a candle flame, or a mantra. This practice helps to calm the mind and improve concentration (Goyal et al., 2014). On the other hand, loving-kindness meditation involves cultivating feelings of compassion and love toward yourself and others. This practice can enhance emotional well-being and foster a sense of connection (Hofmann et al., 2011). Body scan meditation is another effective technique, where you mentally scan your body from head to toe, noticing any areas of tension or discomfort. This practice promotes relaxation and body awareness, helping you to release physical and mental stress (Kabat-Zinn, 1994).

Starting meditation doesn't have to be complicated. Many resources are available, from YouTube videos to apps that guide you through various practices. Set up a comfortable and quiet session space, free from distractions. Use props like mats, pillows, and blankets for support, making it easier to stay relaxed during meditation. Start with short sessions, such as five to ten minutes, and gradually increase the duration as you become more comfortable with the practices. Consistency is paramount, so try to incorporate meditation into your routine, even if it's just for a few minutes each day.

### 9.4 The Importance of Sleep and Hydration

Imagine waking up each morning feeling refreshed and ready to take on the day. Quality sleep is the key to this feeling. When you get a good night's sleep, your brain works better. It helps you think clearly, remember things, and make decisions. Sleep also plays a big role in how you feel. If you sleep well, you're more likely to be in a good mood and handle stress better. Your body uses sleep time to repair muscles, tissues, and cells, which is crucial for physical recovery, especially after exercise (Walker, 2017). Additionally, sleep boosts your immune system, helping you fight off illnesses (National Sleep Foundation, 2020).

To improve sleep quality, start by establishing a regular sleep schedule. Go to bed and wake up at the same time every day of the week, even on weekends, to help regulate your body's internal clock. Creating a relaxing bedtime routine can signal your body that it's time to wind down. Consider activities like reading, calming music, or a warm bath. Avoid caffeine and heavy meals before bed, as they can interfere with your ability to fall asleep. Ensure your sleep environment is comfortable, including a supportive mattress, cozy pillows, and a cool, dark room (Harvard Medical School, 2021).

Staying hydrated is just as important as getting enough sleep. Water is essential for nearly every function in your body. It helps regulate your temperature, keeps your joints lubricated, and aids digestion (Popkin et al., 2010). Proper hydration ensures that your organs and systems work smoothly. Dehydration can lead to issues like headaches, dizziness, and fatigue. Moreover, staying hydrated supports your energy levels, making it easier to stay active and engaged throughout the day.

Keep a water bottle handy throughout the day to stay hydrated. Consistently sipping water can prevent dehydration. Make it a habit to drink a glass of water with each meal to help with hydration and digestion. Water-rich fruits and vegetables, such as cucumbers, oranges, and watermelon, can also boost your hydration levels. Setting reminders on your phone or using apps designed to track water intake can be helpful, especially if you find it challenging to remember to drink water regularly (Armstrong, 2012).

Staying well-hydrated and getting quality sleep are foundational elements of good health, especially as we age. They support cognitive function, boost mood, promote physical recovery, and strengthen your immune system. Simple habits like maintaining a regular sleep schedule, creating a peaceful bedtime routine, and keeping a water bottle close can significantly affect how you feel each day.

## 9.5 Building a Supportive Community

Imagine a vibrant, sunny afternoon where you're surrounded by friends, laughing and sharing stories. This sense of belonging and connection is invaluable, especially as we age. Having a supportive community offers emotional support during tough times and encourages healthy behaviors that can significantly improve your quality of life. A strong network reduces feelings of isolation, which is crucial because loneliness can have profound health implications. Research has shown that social isolation and loneliness are associated with a higher risk of health conditions such as heart disease, stroke, and dementia (Holt-Lunstad, 2015). When you're part of a community, you feel a sense of belonging, enhancing your overall well-being.

Creating and maintaining supportive relationships may seem daunting, but there are many ways to build a community. Joining local clubs or groups tailored to your interests is a great start. Whether it's a book club, a gardening group, or a walking club, these gatherings provide opportunities to meet like-minded individuals. Participating in community events, such as festivals, workshops, or local fairs, can also help you connect with others. Volunteering is another excellent way to build relationships. Not only do you contribute to your community, but you also meet people who share your values and interests. Social media and online forums can also be valuable tools for finding and maintaining connections, especially if mobility or transportation is an issue (Cornwell & Waite, 2009).

Family and friends play a vital role in your support network. Their encouragement and motivation can make a significant difference in achieving your health goals. Sharing activities, like cooking together, going for walks, or attending fitness classes, strengthen these bonds and make the journey to better health more enjoyable. During challenging times, their emotional support is invaluable. They provide a shoulder to lean on and help you navigate difficulties, ensuring you don't have to face them alone.

Community-building activities offer fun and engaging ways to connect with others. Group exercise classes, such as yoga, Tai Chi, or water aerobics, keep you fit and provide a social outlet. Book clubs allow you to share your thoughts and insights on multiple topics, stimulating your mind and fostering meaningful conversations with people. Cooking and gardening groups are both educational and enjoyable as you learn new skills and share delicious, healthy recipes and gardening tips. Social gatherings and potlucks are excellent opportunities to enjoy good food and company, strengthen community ties, and create lasting memories.

These interactions enrich life and offer a sense of purpose and belonging. They remind you that you're part of a community where you're valued and supported. Building and maintaining a supportive community enhances your emotional and physical well-being, making your daily life more fulfilling and joyful.

### 9.6 Tracking Progress: Tools and Tips

Progress tracking is like having a roadmap for your health journey. Tracking motivates you because you can see how far you've come. Knowing you've walked an extra mile this month compared to last can be incredibly encouraging. When you monitor your progress, it also allows for adjustments. Tweak your routine if you find that a particular exercise isn't giving you the desired results. It's just like cooking—you taste and adjust as you go. Tracking improvements over time boosts your confidence and helps you celebrate achievements, making the journey enjoyable and fulfilling.

There are various tools you can use to keep track of your progress. Fitness apps are a great place to start. They can track your steps, monitor your heart rate, and even coach you through workouts. Using journals and planners is an excellent option. You can provide valuable insights by writing down your daily activities, meals, and feelings. Wearable fitness trackers, like Fitbits or Apple Watches, offer real-time data on your physical activities and can even monitor your sleep patterns (Doherty et al., 2017). Online progress charts can also be beneficial, especially if you enjoy visual representations of your achievements.

To track your progress effectively, set specific, measurable goals. Instead of saying, "I want to get fit," aim for "I want to walk 10,000 steps a day." Record your daily activities and achievements in your chosen tracking tool. Consistency is vital, whether it's an app, a journal, or a fitness tracker. Checking your progress helps to keep you on track. Weekly or monthly reviews point out patterns and trends. When you need to catch up on your step count, you can adjust how you walk each day to provide more steps. You may need to take an evening walk or incorporate more activity into your daily routine. Making adjustments based on data ensures that your efforts align with your goals.

Reflecting on your progress significantly boosts your motivation and commitment. Reviewing your achievements, you can identify patterns and trends. You may perform better when you exercise in the morning or find that certain foods give you more energy. Recognizing areas for improvement allows you to fine-tune your approach. Celebrating milestones, no matter how small, reinforces positive behaviors. Did you complete your first 5k walk? Celebrate it! These small victories keep you motivated and committed to your long-term health goals.

By tracking your progress, you create a feedback loop that helps you stay on course. It's a way to hold yourself accountable and ensure you move in the right direction. Plus, there's nothing quite like the satisfaction of seeing your hard work pay off. Whether you're using an app, a journal, or a fitness tracker, the key is to make it a habit. Regular tracking and reflection keep you motivated and make the journey to better health more enjoyable and rewarding.

## 9.7 Inspiring Success Stories

Consider the story of Margaret, a 70-year-old who struggled with obesity and limited mobility. Margaret accepted her weight and health issues as inevitable parts of aging but wondered if there was a better way. She started her change when she tried a low-carb diet inspired by a friend's success. She started slowly by eliminating processed foods and incorporating lean proteins and fats into her meals. Besides these dietary changes, Margaret began a gentle exercise routine with short walks around her neighborhood. Challenges abounded as she started to make changes, such as joint pain and lack of energy, but she continued to push forward.

Margaret's journey was challenging. Initially, she struggled to break old habits and adapt to new ones. Her support system played a crucial role. Margaret's family encouraged her by walking with her each evening and joining her in preparing healthy meals. Gradually, Margaret noticed improvements. She lost weight, her mobility increased, and she felt more energetic. These changes motivated her to continue, and she eventually incorporated strength training and yoga into her routine. Her health improvements didn't stop there. Research has shown that dietary changes combined with physical activity can significantly enhance cognitive function and mood, making Margaret's experience a testament to the power of lifestyle changes (Erickson et al., 2011).

Another inspiring story is that of John, a 68-year-old retired teacher with chronic back pain. His sedentary lifestyle exacerbated his condition, making everyday activities a struggle. John decided to take control of his health after a harrowing episode landed him in the hospital. He started with a physical therapist, who introduced him to low-impact exercises and stretches to relieve his back pain. John also revamped his diet, focusing on anti-inflammatory foods like fatty meats, fatty fish, and nuts. This holistic approach worked wonders for him. Research supports the benefits of an anti-inflammatory diet and exercise in reducing chronic pain and improving quality of life in older adults (Calder, 2013).

John's initial health conditions were daunting, but his determination saw him through. He faced numerous setbacks, including flare-ups of his back pain that made it difficult to stay active. However, his support network, including his wife and friends, provided the encouragement he needed. They joined him in his new routines, making the process enjoyable and less isolating. Over time, John's pain diminished, his mobility improved, and he even regained the ability to engage in activities he once loved, like gardening and playing with his grandchildren.

These stories highlight the profound impact of diet and exercise on seniors' lives. Margaret and John experienced increased independence, allowing them to enjoy activities they had previously given up on. Their quality of life improved significantly, with enhanced social connections and a renewed sense of purpose. The confidence they gained from their health improvements radiated into other areas of their lives, making them more active and engaged members of their communities.

The key takeaway from these stories is the power of persistence and consistency. Both Margaret and John faced significant challenges but overcame them through steady, incremental changes. Their success underscores the importance of a strong support network. Whether it's family, friends, or a community group, having people who encourage and motivate you can make a difference. Setting realistic goals was also crucial. They didn't aim for drastic changes overnight but focused on small, achievable steps leading to significant progress. Finally, celebrating small victories helped them stay motivated and committed to their health journeys.

### 9.8 Staying Motivated: Long-Term Health and Wellness

Maintaining long-term motivation can be challenging. Initially, you might feel enthusiastic and driven, but that excitement can wane over time. Plateaus and setbacks can also dampen your spirits. You might find your progress stalling or face unexpected obstacles that make it hard to stay on track. Distractions and life changes, such as family commitments or health issues, can further complicate your efforts. It's easy to lose sight of your goals when life gets in the way, making it crucial to find ways to keep motivation alive.

One effective strategy for maintaining motivation is setting new and varied goals and introducing new challenges to keep things moving forward instead of sticking to the same routine. You could aim to walk a little further each week or try a new exercise like swimming or Tai Chi. Studies have shown that setting specific, challenging goals can significantly enhance motivation and adherence to exercise programs (Locke & Latham, 2002). Finding activities you genuinely enjoy can make a big difference. When exercise feels like play rather than work, you're more likely to stick with it. Regularly reviewing your progress can also be motivating. Take time to reflect on your achievements and set new targets based on your progress. Seeking continuous education and inspiration through books, podcasts, YouTube videos, or online courses can provide fresh perspectives and keep you engaged.

A positive mindset is essential for long-term success. Embrace a growth mindset, where you view challenges as opportunities to learn and grow rather than setbacks. Focus on progress, not perfection. Every step forward, no matter how small, is a victory. Practice self-compassion, acknowledging that everyone has off days and that it's okay to stumble. Celebrating big and small achievements reinforces positive behavior and keeps you motivated. Whether it's completing a month of regular exercise or simply feeling more energetic, take time to celebrate your successes.

Numerous resources are available to help keep your motivation high. Inspirational books and podcasts can provide valuable insights and encouragement. Online health communities offer a platform to share experiences, seek advice, and locate support. Fitness challenges and programs can add structure and excitement to your routine. Support groups and coaching provide personalized guidance and accountability, helping you stay on track even when motivation wanes.

To summarize, staying motivated over the long term requires various strategies. Setting new goals, finding enjoyable activities, regularly reviewing progress, and seeking continuous inspiration are all vital. A positive mindset, focusing on growth and celebrating achievements, can keep you going. Use resources like books, online communities, and support groups to maintain enthusiasm and commitment.

## Help Others Get Healthy and Active

Now that you have all the tools to **improve your health and strengthen your body**, it's time to share your journey and help others find the same support.

By leaving a review on Amazon, you'll show other **seniors** exactly where they can get the information they need to feel stronger and more active, just like you. Your words will inspire others to start their own path toward **getting healthy through diet and exercise**.

Thank you for helping to keep the **journey to better health** alive. By sharing your experience, you're helping others—and together, we're building a community of healthier, happier seniors.

Scan the QR code to leave your review on Amazon.

# Conclusion

As we come to the end of this journey together, I am restating the primary purpose and vision of this book. This book aims to provide you with a comprehensive diet and exercise guide specifically tailored for seniors. I have tried to empower you to build strength, balance, flexibility, and mental well-being, paving the way for a fulfilling and active life throughout your golden years. At 55, I understand firsthand the importance of maintaining a healthy lifestyle as I age, and I hope my passion for senior wellness has resonated with you.

A foundational principle emphasized is the importance of prioritizing diet. You must start here. Achieving metabolic health through proper nutrition lays the groundwork for any successful exercise routine. Exploration of unconventional diets like Keto, Carnivore, and Paleo, backed by the insights of leading experts such as Dr. Shawn Baker, Dr. Ken Berry, and Dr. Annette Bosworth, shows how each can be useful in this journey (Baker, 2019; Berry, 2020; Bosworth, 2019). These diets can help you lose weight, control blood sugar and blood pressure, and enhance mental strength. Once you have begun the journey to losing weight and taming the inflammation in your body, it becomes infinitely easier to embrace an active lifestyle. Remember, making small, consistent dietary changes can significantly improve your health.

We also delved into various exercise routines and techniques, providing a diverse toolkit to keep your workouts engaging and effective. We've tried to cover everything from walking and chair exercises to strength training and balance exercises (Taylor et al., 2004). We introduced you to the benefits of Tai Chi and yoga and even explored advanced techniques like blood flow restriction training, vibration plates, and aquatic exercises (Anderson & Taylor, 2011). Each activity offers unique advantages, and incorporating various exercises ensures a well-rounded fitness routine.

But our approach goes beyond just physical activity. A holistic approach to health connects the body, mind, and emotions. We discussed the importance of stress reduction techniques, such as deep breathing and mindfulness meditation, and how they can improve overall well-being (Kabat-Zinn, 2003). We also emphasized the critical roles of sleep and hydration in maintaining good health (Hirshkowitz et al., 2015). Building a supportive community is another key aspect of this holistic approach. Surrounding yourself with family, friends, and like-minded individuals can provide the encouragement and motivation you need to stay on track.

Here are some key takeaways to keep in mind:

1. **Prioritize Diet:** Achieving metabolic health through a well-balanced diet is crucial before starting an exercise routine.

2. **Diverse Exercise Routine:** Incorporate various exercises, such as walking, chair exercises, strength training, and balance exercises, to keep your workouts engaging and ever-changing.
3. **Holistic Health:** Enhances your overall well-being, focusing on stress reduction, mind-body exercises, quality sleep, hydration, and building a supportive community.

Now, it's time for action. I encourage you to take the first step towards a healthier lifestyle by making small, manageable changes in your diet and exercise routines. Set realistic goals and stay committed to your health journey. Remember, it's the small, consistent efforts that lead to significant improvements.

Don't stop here. Continue learning about health and fitness, stay updated with new research, and adapt your daily routines to keep progressing. The field of health and wellness is ever-evolving, and staying informed will help you make the best choices for your well-being.

Building and maintaining a supportive community is essential, so contact family, friends, and local or online groups for support and encouragement. Share your journey with others, and you'll find that the sense of community can be a powerful motivator.

Remember the inspiring success stories we've shared throughout this book. Individuals like Margaret and John faced significant challenges but achieved remarkable health improvements through persistence and dedication (Erickson et al., 2011). Believe in your potential to achieve similar results. Your journey may be unique, but diet, exercise, and holistic health principles are universal.

Finally, I want to leave you with an empowering thought: Making positive changes is always possible. Every step toward a healthier lifestyle is a step toward a more fulfilling and active life. Embrace this journey with an open heart and mind, celebrate each milestone, and look forward to your next adventure.

Thank you for allowing me to be a part of your health journey. Here's to a healthier, happier, and more vibrant you!

# References

**Introduction References**

Baker, S. (2019). *The Carnivore Diet*. Victory Belt Publishing.

Berry, K. (2019). *Lies My Doctor Told Me: Medical Myths That Can Harm Your Health*. Victory Belt Publishing.

Bosworth, A. (2020). *KetoContinuum: Consistently Keto for Life*. BozMD Publishing.

Centers for Disease Control and Prevention. (2013). *The state of aging and health in America 2013*. Retrieved from https://www.cdc.gov/aging/pdf/state-aging-health-in-america-2013.pdf

National Cholesterol Education Program (NCEP) Expert Panel on Detection, Evaluation, and Treatment of High Blood Cholesterol in Adults (Adult Treatment Panel III). (2002). *Third report of the National Cholesterol Education Program (NCEP) expert panel on detection, evaluation, and treatment of high blood cholesterol in adults (Adult Treatment Panel III) final report.*

**Chapter 1 Section 1.1**

Appel, L. J., Moore, T. J., Obarzanek, E., Vollmer, W. M., Svetkey, L. P., Sacks, F. M., ... & Harsha, D. W. (1997). A clinical trial of the effects of dietary patterns on blood pressure. *The New England Journal of Medicine, 336*(16), 1117-1124.

Calder, P. C. (2020). Nutrition, immunity, and COVID-19. *BMJ Nutrition, Prevention & Health, 3*(1), 74-92.

Feinman, R. D., Pogozelski, W. K., Astrup, A., Bernstein, R. K., Fine, E. J., Westman, E. C., ... & Volek, J. S. (2015). Dietary carbohydrate restriction as the first approach in diabetes management: Critical review and evidence base. *Nutrition, 31*(1), 1-13.

Kerksick, C. M., Wilborn, C. D., Roberts, M. D., Smith-Ryan, A., Kleiner, S. M., Jäger, R., ... & Kreider, R. B. (2017). ISSN exercise & sports nutrition review update: Research & recommendations. *Journal of the International Society of Sports Nutrition, 15*(1), 38.

Lustig, R. H., Schmidt, L. A., & Brindis, C. D. (2016). Public health: The toxic truth about sugar. *Nature, 482*(7383), 27-29.

Messier, S. P., Gutekunst, D. J., Davis, C., & DeVita, P. (2013). Weight loss reduces knee-joint loads in overweight and obese older adults with knee osteoarthritis. *Arthritis & Rheumatism, 61*(5), 640-650.

Monteiro, C. A., Cannon, G., Moubarac, J. C., Levy, R. B., Louzada, M. L. C., &

Jaime, P. C. (2018). The UN decade of nutrition, the NOVA food classification and the trouble with ultra-processing. *Public Health Nutrition, 21*(1), 5-17.

Phillips, S. M. (2017). Current concepts and unresolved questions in dietary protein requirements and supplements in adults. *Frontiers in Nutrition, 4*, 13.

Westman, E. C., Yancy, W. S., Mavropoulos, J. C., Marquart, M., & McDuffie, J. R. (2018). The effect of a low-carbohydrate, ketogenic diet versus a low-glycemic index diet on glycemic control in type 2 diabetes mellitus. *Nutrition & Metabolism, 5*(1), 36.

Yehuda, S., Rabinovitz, S., & Mostofsky, D. I. (1999). Essential fatty acids are mediators of brain biochemistry and cognitive functions. *The Journal of Neuroscience Research, 56*(5), 565-570.

**References 1.2**

DeFronzo, R. A. (2009). From the triumvirate to the ominous octet: a new paradigm for the treatment of type 2 diabetes mellitus. *Diabetes, 58*(4), 773-795.

Ford, E. S., Zhao, G., Li, C., & Pearson, W. S. (2010). Trends in obesity and abdominal obesity among adults in the United States from 1999-2008. *International Journal of Obesity, 35*(5), 736-743.

Gerstein, H. C., Miller, M. E., Byington, R. P., Goff, D. C., Bigger, J. T., Buse, J. B., ... & Genuth, S. (2008). Effects of intensive glucose lowering in type 2 diabetes. *The New England Journal of Medicine, 358*(24), 2545-2559.

Goldstein, L. B., Adams, R., Becker, K., Furberg, C. D., Gorelick, P. B., Hademenos, G., ... & Stroke Council of the American Heart Association. (2009). Primary prevention of ischemic stroke: A statement for healthcare professionals from the Stroke Council of the American Heart Association. *Circulation, 103*(1), 163-182.

Grundy, S. M. (2016). Recent advances in cholesterol-lowering therapy: Mechanisms and opportunities. *Cell Metabolism, 23*(2), 219-226.

Gunstad, J., Paul, R. H., Cohen, R. A., Tate, D. F., Spitznagel, M. B., & Gordon, E. (2007). Elevated body mass index is associated with executive dysfunction in otherwise healthy adults. *Comprehensive Psychiatry, 48*(1), 57-61.

Hotamisligil, G. S. (2006). Inflammation and metabolic disorders. *Nature, 444*(7121), 860-867.

Phinney, S. D., & Volek, J. S. (2011). *The Art and Science of Low Carbohydrate Living: An Expert Guide to Making the Life-Saving Benefits of Carbohydrate Restriction Sustainable and Enjoyable*. Beyond Obesity LLC.

Phillips, S. M. (2017). Current concepts and unresolved questions in dietary protein requirements and supplements in adults. *Frontiers in Nutrition, 4*, 13.

Sawka, M. N., Cheuvront, S. N., & Kenefick, R. W. (2007). Hypohydration and human performance: impact of environment and physiological mechanisms. *Sports Medicine, 37*(10), 909-923.

Van Cauter, E., Leproult, R., & Plat, L. (2008). Age-related changes in slow-wave sleep and REM sleep and relationship with growth hormone and cortisol levels in healthy men. *JAMA, 284*(7), 861-868.

Westman, E. C., Yancy, W. S., Mavropoulos, J. C., Marquart, M., & McDuffie, J. R. (2018). The effect of a low-carbohydrate, ketogenic diet versus a low-glycemic index diet on glycemic control in type 2 diabetes mellitus. *Nutrition & Metabolism, 5*(1), 36.

**References 1.3**

Breen, L., & Phillips, S. M. (2011). Skeletal muscle protein metabolism in the elderly: Interventions to counteract the 'anabolic resistance' of ageing. *Nutrition & Metabolism, 8*(1), 68.

Eaton, S. B., Konner, M., & Shostak, M. (1988). Stone agers in the fast lane: Chronic degenerative diseases in evolutionary perspective. *American Journal of Medicine, 84*(4), 739-749.

Harman, D. (2003). The free radical theory of aging. *Antioxidants & Redox Signaling, 5*(5), 557-561.

Henrotin, Y., Lambert, C., Couchourel, D., Ripoll, C., & Chiotelli, E. (2011). Nutraceuticals: Do they represent a new era in the management of osteoarthritis? A narrative review from the lessons taken with five products. *Osteoarthritis and Cartilage, 19*(1), 1-21.

Joseph, J. A., Shukitt-Hale, B., & Casadesus, G. (2009). Reversing the deleterious effects of aging on neuronal communication and behavior: Beneficial properties of fruit polyphenolic compounds. *American Journal of Clinical Nutrition, 81*(1), 313S-316S.

Lanham-New, S. A., et al. (2012). Calcium and vitamin D. *Nutrition & Health, 2*(1), 113-124.

Malik, V. S., Schulze, M. B., & Hu, F. B. (2010). Intake of sugar-sweetened beverages and weight gain: A systematic review. *The American Journal of Clinical Nutrition, 84*(2), 274-288.

Mozaffarian, D., & Wu, J. H. Y. (2011). Omega-3 fatty acids and cardiovascular disease: Effects on risk factors, molecular pathways, and clinical events. *Journal of the American College of Cardiology, 58*(20), 2047-2067.

**References 1.4**

American College of Sports Medicine. (2011). *ACSM's guidelines for exercise testing and prescription* (8th ed.). Lippincott Williams & Wilkins.

Berry, K. (2018). *Lies my doctor told me: Medical myths that can harm your health.* Victory Belt Publishing.

Breen, L., & Phillips, S. M. (2011). Skeletal muscle protein metabolism in the elderly: Interventions to counteract the 'anabolic resistance' of ageing. *Nutrition & Metabolism, 8*(1), 68.

de la Monte, S. M., & Wands, J. R. (2008). Alzheimer's disease is type 3 diabetes—evidence reviewed. *Journal of Diabetes Science and Technology, 2*(6), 1101-1113.

Nelson, M. E., Rejeski, W. J., Blair, S. N., Duncan, P. W., Judge, J. O., King, A. C., ... & Castaneda-Sceppa, C. (2004). Physical activity and public health in older adults: Recommendation from the American College of Sports Medicine and the American Heart Association. *Medicine & Science in Sports & Exercise, 36*(11), 1997-2003.

Siri-Tarino, P. W., Sun, Q., Hu, F. B., & Krauss, R. M. (2010). Meta-analysis of prospective cohort studies evaluating the association of saturated fat with cardiovascular disease. *The American Journal of Clinical Nutrition, 91*(3), 535-546.

Warburton, D. E., Nicol, C. W., & Bredin, S. S. (2006). Health benefits of physical activity: The evidence. *CMAJ, 174*(6), 801-809.

Westman, E. C. (2002). Is dietary carbohydrate essential for human nutrition? *American Journal of Clinical Nutrition, 75*(5), 951-953.

**References 1.5**

American Heart Association. (2017). Understanding blood pressure readings. Retrieved from https://www.heart.org/en/health-topics/high-blood-pressure/understanding-blood-pressure-readings

Bandura, A. (1997). *Self-efficacy: The exercise of control.* W.H. Freeman.

Locke, E. A., & Latham, G. P. (2002). Building a practically useful theory of goal setting and task motivation: A 35-year odyssey. *American Psychologist, 57*(9), 705–717.

National Institutes of Health. (2016). *Your guide to lowering blood pressure with DASH.* U.S. Department of Health and Human Services.

**Chapter 2 References**

**References 2.1**

Boden, G., Sargrad, K., Homko, C., Mozzoli, M., & Stein, T. P. (2005). Effect of a low-carbohydrate diet on appetite, blood glucose levels, and insulin resistance in obese patients with type 2 diabetes. *Annals of Internal Medicine, 142*(6), 403-411. https://doi.org/10.7326/0003-4819-142-6-200503150-00006

Bueno, N. B., de Melo, I. S. V., de Oliveira, S. L., & da Rocha Ataide, T. (2013). Very-low-carbohydrate ketogenic diet v. low-fat diet for long-term weight loss: A meta-analysis of randomised controlled trials. *British Journal of Nutrition, 110*(7), 1178-1187. https://doi.org/10.1017/S0007114513000548

Cunnane, S. C., Courchesne-Loyer, A., Vandenberghe, C., St-Pierre, V., Fortier, M., Hennebelle, M., ... & Castellano, C. A. (2016). Can ketones compensate for deteriorating brain glucose uptake during aging? Implications for the risk and treatment of Alzheimer's disease. *Annals of the New York Academy of Sciences, 1367*(1), 12-20. https://doi.org/10.1111/nyas.12999

Paoli, A., Rubini, A., Volek, J. S., & Grimaldi, K. A. (2013). Beyond weight loss: A review of the therapeutic uses of very-low-carbohydrate (ketogenic) diets. *European Journal of Clinical Nutrition, 67*(8), 789-796. https://doi.org/10.1038/ejcn.2013.116

Taylor, M. K., Sullivan, D. K., Mahnken, J. D., Burns, J. M., & Swerdlow, R. H. (2018). Feasibility and efficacy data from a ketogenic diet intervention in Alzheimer's disease. *Alzheimer's & Dementia: Translational Research & Clinical Interventions, 4,* 28-36. https://doi.org/10.1016/j.trci.2017.11.002

Westman, E. C., Mavropoulos, J. C., Yancy, W. S., & Volek, J. S. (2003). A review of low-carbohydrate ketogenic diets. *Current Atherosclerosis Reports, 5*(6), 476-483. https://doi.org/10.1007/s11883-003-0048-7

American Dietetic Association. (2009). Dietary guidelines for Americans.

Johnston, C. A., Stevens, B., & Foreyt, J. P. (2014). Strategies for healthy weight loss: from vitamin C to the glycemic response. Journal of the American College of Nutrition, 33(3), 176-183.

Santos, I., Vieira, P. N., Silva, M. N., Sardinha, L. B., & Teixeira, P. J. (2017). Perceived barriers and facilitators of physical activity: What really matters to patients with diabetes? International Journal of Behavioral Nutrition and Physical Activity, 14, 79.

Volek, J. S., & Phinney, S. D. (2012). The Art and Science of Low Carbohydrate Living: An Expert Guide to Making the Life-Saving Benefits of Carbohydrate Restriction Sustainable and Enjoyable.

Zimmerman, M. (2017). The role of social support in diet and exercise. Journal of Health Psychology, 22(6), 752-762.

**References 2.2**

Baker, S. (2019). *The Carnivore Diet*. Victory Belt Publishing.

Mikovits, J., & Heckenlively, K. (2020). *Plague of Corruption: Restoring Faith in the Promise of Science*. Skyhorse Publishing.

Naiman, P. (2019). *Diet Doctor: The Carnivore Diet Guide*. Retrieved from https://www.dietdoctor.com

Norris, M. (2020). Carnivore diet: Benefits, drawbacks, and everything you need to know. *Healthline*. Retrieved from https://www.healthline.com

Smith, D., & Hiltz, A. (2018). Cognitive enhancement through dietary strategies. *Nutrition and Aging, 5*(1), 25-34.

Volek, J. S., & Phinney, S. D. (2011). *The Art and Science of Low Carbohydrate Living: An Expert Guide to Making the Life-Saving Benefits of Carbohydrate Restriction Sustainable and Enjoyable*. Beyond Obesity LLC.

**References 2.3**

Cordain, L. (2011). *The Paleo Diet: Lose Weight and Get Healthy by Eating the Foods You Were Designed to Eat*. Wiley.

Cordain, L., & Friel, J. (2005). *The Paleo Diet for Athletes: A Nutritional Formula for Peak Athletic Performance.* Rodale Books.

Sisson, M. (2011). *The Primal Blueprint: Reprogram your genes for effortless weight loss, vibrant health, and boundless energy.* Primal Nutrition.

Wolf, R. (2010). *The Paleo Solution: The Original Human Diet.* Victory Belt Publishing.

These references support the claims about the benefits of the Paleo diet, providing insights from experts and scientific literature regarding the advantages of following this dietary approach.

**References 2.4**

Baker, S. (2019). *The Carnivore Diet.* Victory Belt Publishing.

Cordain, L. (2010). *The Paleo Diet: Lose Weight and Get Healthy by Eating the Foods You Were Designed to Eat.* Wiley.

Westman, E. C., Phinney, S. D., & Volek, J. S. (2007). *The New Atkins for a New You: The Ultimate Diet for Shedding Weight and Feeling Great.* Simon and Schuster.

**References 2.5**

Berry, K. (2019). *Lies My Doctor Told Me.* Victory Belt Publishing.

Bosworth, A. (2020). *KetoContinuum: Consistently Keto for Life.* Dr. Boz.

Chaffee, A. (2021). *Nutritional Wisdom.* Self-published.

Westman, E. C., Phinney, S. D., & Volek, J. S. (2007). *The New Atkins for a New You: The Ultimate Diet for Shedding Weight and Feeling Great.* Simon & Schuster.

**Chapter 3 References**

**References 3.1**

Baker, S. (2019). *The Carnivore Diet.* Victory Belt Publishing.

MeatRx. (n.d.). About MeatRx. Retrieved from https://meatrx.com

Revero Health. (n.d.). Revero Health: Personalized healthcare for metabolic and autoimmune conditions. Retrieved from https://revero.com

**References 3.2**

Berry, K. (2017). *Lies My Doctor Told Me: Medical Myths That Can Harm Your Health.* Victory Belt Publishing.

Berry, K. (n.d.). *Dr. Ken Berry MD.* Retrieved from https://www.drberry.com

**References 3.3**

Westman, E. C., Berger, A., & Thole, M. (2020). *End Your Carb Confusion: A Simple Guide to Customize Your Carb Intake for Optimal Health.* Victory Belt Publishing.

Westman, E. C., Phinney, S. D., & Volek, J. S. (2014). *Keto Clarity: Your Definitive Guide to the Benefits of a Low-Carb, High-Fat Diet.* Victory Belt Publishing.

Westman, E. C., Yancy, W. S., Mavropoulos, J. C., Marquart, M., & McDuffie, J. R. (2008). The effect of a low-carbohydrate, ketogenic diet versus a low-glycemic index diet on glycemic control in type 2 diabetes mellitus. *Nutrition & Metabolism, 5*(36). https://doi.org/10.1186/1743-7075-5-36

## References 3.4

Bosworth, A. (2020). *KetoContinuum: Consistently keto for life.* BozMD Publishing.

Chrousos, G. P. (2009). Stress and disorders of the stress system. *Nature Reviews Endocrinology, 5*(7), 374-381.

Mattson, M. P., Longo, V. D., & Harvie, M. (2017). Impact of intermittent fasting on health and disease processes. *Ageing Research Reviews, 39,* 46-58.

Walker, M. (2017). *Why we sleep: Unlocking the power of sleep and dreams.* Scribner.

## References 3.5

Chaffee, A. (2023). *Nutritional Strategies for Optimal Health.* [Details based on actual publication].

## References Chapter 4.1

Academy of Nutrition and Dietetics. (2023). **Meal planning basics**. https://www.eatright.org/food/planning-and-prep

Cleveland Clinic. (2023). **Understanding healthy fats**. https://health.clevelandclinic.org/understanding-healthy-fats/

Cordain, L. (2010). **The Paleo diet: Lose weight and get healthy by eating the foods you were designed to eat**. Wiley.

Harvard Medical School. (2022). **Keto diet: A beginner's guide to low carb eating**. https://www.health.harvard.edu/blog/keto-diet-a-beginners-guide-202201242682

Harvard T.H. Chan School of Public Health. (n.d.). **The nutrition source**. https://www.hsph.harvard.edu/nutritionsource/

Mayo Clinic. (2023). **Meal planning: A route to a healthier diet**. https://www.mayoclinic.org

## References 4.2

American Heart Association. (2019). **Fish and omega-3 fatty acids**. https://www.heart.org

Harvard T.H. Chan School of Public Health. (n.d.). **The nutrition source**. https://www.hsph.harvard.edu/nutritionsource/

Mayo Clinic. (2022). **Nutrient-dense foods and the senior diet**. https://www.mayoclinic.org

National Institute on Aging. (2021). **Healthy eating as you age**. https://www.nia.nih.gov

U.S. Department of Agriculture. (2020). **Dietary guidelines for Americans 2020-2025**. https://www.dietaryguidelines.gov

## References 4.3

American Heart Association. (2020). **Salmon and omega-3 fatty acids**. https://www.heart.org

Harvard T.H. Chan School of Public Health. (n.d.). **The nutrition source: Low-carb diets**. https://www.hsph.harvard.edu/nutritionsource/

Mayo Clinic. (2021). **Low-carb and ketogenic diets.** https://www.mayoclinic.org

Perfect Keto. (2022). **Easy keto recipes for beginners.** https://www.perfectketo.com

**References 4.4**

Carnivore Aurelius. (2022). **Carnivore diet: Meal ideas and recipes.** https://www.carnivoreaurelius.com

Harvard T.H. Chan School of Public Health. (n.d.). **The nutrition source: Grass-fed vs. conventional beef.** https://www.hsph.harvard.edu/nutritionsource/

Peterson, S. (2020). **The carnivore diet for beginners: Simple recipes to boost energy.** Victory Belt Publishing.

Saladino, P. (2020). **The carnivore code: Unlocking the secrets to optimal health by returning to our ancestral diet.** Mariner Books.

Sisson, M. (2021). **The primal blueprint: Reprogram your genes for effortless weight loss, vibrant health, and boundless energy.** Primal Nutrition.

**References 4.5**

Ballantyne, S. (2014). **The Paleo approach: Reverse autoimmune disease and heal your body.** Victory Belt Publishing.

Cordain, L. (2011). **The Paleo diet: Lose weight and get healthy by eating the foods you were designed to eat.** Wiley.

Wolf, R. (2016). **The Paleo solution: The original human diet.** Victory Belt Publishing.

**Chapter 5 References**

**References 5.1**

American College of Sports Medicine. (2021). **ACSM's guidelines for exercise testing and prescription** (11th ed.). Lippincott Williams & Wilkins.

American Heart Association. (2021). **Exercise and physical activity in older adults.** https://www.heart.org

Centers for Disease Control and Prevention. (2022). **How much physical activity do older adults need?** https://www.cdc.gov/physicalactivity/basics/older_adults/

Mayo Clinic. (2021). **Exercise: A guide to getting started.** https://www.mayoclinic.org

**References 5.2-5.3**

American College of Sports Medicine. (2021). **ACSM's guidelines for exercise testing and prescription** (11th ed.). Lippincott Williams & Wilkins.

American Heart Association. (2021). **Walking for heart health.** https://www.heart.org

Harvard Health Publishing. (2020). **The importance of warm-up and cool-down exercises.** https://www.health.harvard.edu

Mayo Clinic. (2021). **Exercise and the importance of warming up and cooling down**. https://www.mayoclinic.org

**References 5.4-5.5**

American College of Sports Medicine. (2021). **ACSM's guidelines for exercise testing and prescription** (11th ed.). Lippincott Williams & Wilkins.

Harvard Health Publishing. (2020). **Flexibility exercises for seniors: Stretching safely**. https://www.health.harvard.edu

Mayo Clinic. (2021). **Chair exercises and stretching: Staying fit with limited mobility**. https://www.mayoclinic.org

**References Chapter 6 6.1**

American College of Sports Medicine. (2021). **ACSM's guidelines for exercise testing and prescription** (11th ed.). Lippincott Williams & Wilkins.

Centers for Disease Control and Prevention. (2023). **Falls among older adults: An overview**. https://www.cdc.gov/falls/facts.html

Johns Hopkins Medicine. (2021). **Fall prevention and older adults**. https://www.hopkinsmedicine.org

**References 6.2-6.3**

American College of Sports Medicine. (2021). **ACSM's guidelines for exercise testing and prescription** (11th ed.). Lippincott Williams & Wilkins.

Harvard Health Publishing. (2020). **Tai Chi and qi gong: Better balance for life**. https://www.health.harvard.edu

Mayo Clinic. (2021). **Balance exercises for older adults**. https://www.mayoclinic.org

**References 6.4-6.5**

American College of Sports Medicine. (2021). **ACSM's guidelines for exercise testing and prescription** (11th ed.). Lippincott Williams & Wilkins.

Harvard Health Publishing. (2021). **Yoga for better balance**. https://www.health.harvard.edu

Iyengar, B. K. S. (2001). **Light on yoga**. Schocken Books.

Mayo Clinic. (2020). **Yoga: A beginner's guide to practice and benefits**. https://www.mayoclinic.org

**References 7-7.1**

American College of Sports Medicine. (2021). **ACSM's guidelines for exercise testing and prescription** (11th ed.). Lippincott Williams & Wilkins.

Harvard Health Publishing. (2019). **Strength training for seniors: How to build muscle safely**. https://www.health.harvard.edu

Mayo Clinic. (2021). **Bodyweight exercises for seniors**. https://www.mayoclinic.org

### References 7.2

American College of Sports Medicine. (2021). ACSM's guidelines for exercise testing and prescription (11th ed.). Lippincott Williams & Wilkins.

Harvard Health Publishing. (2019). Strength training for seniors: How to build muscle safely. https://www.health.harvard.edu

Mayo Clinic. (2021). Strength training: How to build strength safely. https://www.mayoclinic.org

### References 7.3

American College of Sports Medicine. (2021). **ACSM's guidelines for exercise testing and prescription** (11th ed.). Lippincott Williams & Wilkins.

Harvard Health Publishing. (2021). **Strength training for seniors: How to build muscle safely.** https://www.health.harvard.edu

Mayo Clinic. (2021). **Strength training: Get stronger, leaner, healthier.** https://www.mayoclinic.org

### References 7.4-7.5

American College of Sports Medicine. (2021). **ACSM's guidelines for exercise testing and prescription** (11th ed.). Lippincott Williams & Wilkins.

Harvard Health Publishing. (2019). **Strength training for seniors: How to build muscle safely.** https://www.health.harvard.edu

Hughes, L., Paton, B., Rosenblatt, B., Gissane, C., & Patterson, S. D. (2017). Blood flow restriction training in clinical musculoskeletal rehabilitation: A systematic review and meta-analysis. *British Journal of Sports Medicine, 51*(13), 1003-1011.

Loenneke, J. P., Fahs, C. A., Rossow, L. M., & Abe, T. (2016). The anabolic benefits of venous blood flow restriction training may be induced by muscle cell swelling. *Medical Hypotheses, 78*(1), 151-154.

Slysz, J., Stultz, J., & Burr, J. F. (2016). The efficacy of blood flow restricted exercise: A systematic review & meta-analysis. *Journal of Science and Medicine in Sport, 19*(8), 669-675.

American College of Sports Medicine. (2021). **ACSM's guidelines for exercise testing and prescription** (11th ed.). Lippincott Williams & Wilkins.

Harvard Health Publishing. (2019). **Strength training for seniors: How to build muscle safely.** Retrieved from https://www.health.harvard.edu

### References 8-8.1

American College of Sports Medicine. (2021). **ACSM's guidelines for exercise testing and prescription** (11th ed.). Lippincott Williams & Wilkins.

American Heart Association. (2018). **The benefits of aerobic exercise.** https://www.heart.org

Harvard Health Publishing. (2019). **Aerobic exercise: Top 10 reasons to get physical.** https://www.health.harvard.edu

Mayo Clinic. (2021). **Aerobic exercise: How to warm up and cool down.** https://

www.mayoclinic.org

**References 8.2-8.3**

American College of Sports Medicine. (2021). **ACSM's guidelines for exercise testing and prescription** (11th ed.). Lippincott Williams & Wilkins.

Harvard Health Publishing. (2020). **The benefits of low-impact exercise**. https://www.health.harvard.edu

Mayo Clinic. (2021). **Aerobic exercise: How to warm up and cool down**. https://www.mayoclinic.org

**References 8.4**

American College of Sports Medicine. (2021). **ACSM's guidelines for exercise testing and prescription** (11th ed.). Lippincott Williams & Wilkins.

American Heart Association. (2018). **The benefits of aquatic exercise**. https://www.heart.org

Harvard Health Publishing. (2020). **The benefits of low-impact exercise**. https://www.health.harvard.edu

Mayo Clinic. (2021). **Water exercise: Swimming and water workouts**. https://www.mayoclinic.org

**References 8.5**

American College of Sports Medicine. (2021). **ACSM's guidelines for exercise testing and prescription** (11th ed.). Lippincott Williams & Wilkins.

Harvard Health Publishing. (2019). **Staying motivated to exercise: Tips and tricks**. https://www.health.harvard.edu

Locke, E. A., & Latham, G. P. (2002). **Building a practically useful theory of goal setting and task motivation: A 35-year odyssey**. *American Psychologist, 57*(9), 705-717. https://doi.org/10.1037/0003-066X.57.9.705

Mayo Clinic. (2020). **Fitness basics: Elements of a well-rounded exercise routine**. https://www.mayoclinic.org

**References 9-9.1**

Centers for Disease Control and Prevention. (2021). *Physical activity and mental health*. https://www.cdc.gov

Harvard Health Publishing. (2020). *The mental health benefits of exercise: From depression and anxiety to stress*. https://www.health.harvard.edu

Mather, A. S., Rodriguez, C., Guthrie, M. F., McHarg, A. M., Reid, I. C., & McMurdo, M. E. T. (2002). Effects of exercise on depressive symptoms in older adults with poorly responsive depressive disorder: Randomised controlled trial. *American Journal of Geriatric Psychiatry, 10*(4), 467–472. https://doi.org/10.1097/00019442-200207000-00010

National Institute on Aging. (2020). *Exercise and physical activity: Your everyday guide from the National Institute on Aging*. https://www.nia.nih.gov

National Sleep Foundation. (2020). *Exercise and sleep: How physical activity impacts rest.* https://www.sleepfoundation.org

**References 9.2**

American Psychological Association. (2017). *The role of a healthy lifestyle in mental health.* https://www.apa.org

American Psychological Association. (2018). *Stress effects on the body.* https://www.apa.org

Harvard Health Publishing. (2020). *Exercising to relax: Boosting mental health through fitness.* https://www.health.harvard.edu

Jacobson, E. (1938). *Progressive relaxation.* University of Chicago Press.

Kabat-Zinn, J. (1994). *Wherever you go, there you are: Mindfulness meditation in everyday life.* Hyperion.

National Institute of Mental Health. (2021). *Managing stress.* https://www.nimh.nih.gov

Naparstek, B. (1994). *Staying well with guided imagery.* Warner Books.

**References 9.3-9.4**

Armstrong, L. E. (2012). Challenges of linking chronic dehydration and fluid consumption to health outcomes. *Nutrition Reviews, 70*(Suppl 2), S121–S127. https://doi.org/10.1111/j.1753-4887.2012.00520.x

Goyal, M., Singh, S., Sibinga, E. M., Gould, N. F., Rowland-Seymour, A., Sharma, R., & Haythornthwaite, J. A. (2014). Meditation programs for psychological stress and well-being: A systematic review and meta-analysis. *JAMA Internal Medicine, 174*(3), 357–368. https://doi.org/10.1001/jamainternmed.2013.13018

Harvard Health Publishing. (2020). *Mindfulness meditation may ease anxiety, mental stress.* https://www.health.harvard.edu

Harvard Medical School. (2021). *Healthy sleep tips.* https://www.health.harvard.edu

Hofmann, S. G., Grossman, P., & Hinton, D. E. (2011). Loving-kindness and compassion meditation: Potential for psychological interventions. *Clinical Psychology Review, 31*(7), 1126–1132. https://doi.org/10.1016/j.cpr.2011.07.003

Kabat-Zinn, J. (1994). *Wherever you go, there you are: Mindfulness meditation in everyday life.* Hyperion.

National Sleep Foundation. (2020). *How much sleep do you really need?* https://www.sleepfoundation.org

Popkin, B. M., D'Anci, K. E., & Rosenberg, I. H. (2010). Water, hydration, and health. *Nutrition Reviews, 68*(8), 439–458. https://doi.org/10.1111/j.1753-4887.2010.00304.x

Walker, M. (2017). *Why we sleep: Unlocking the power of sleep and dreams.* Scribner.

**References 9.5-9.6**

Cornwell, E. Y., & Waite, L. J. (2009). Social disconnectedness, perceived isolation, and health among older adults. *Journal of Health and Social Behavior, 50*(1), 31-48. https://doi.org/10.1177/002214650905000103

Doherty, A., Jackson, D., Hammerla, N., Ploetz, T., Olivier, P., Granat, M. H., ... & Foster, C. (2017). Wearable sensors: The role of technology in physical activity intervention. *Journal of the American Medical Informatics Association, 24*(1), 118-126. https://doi.org/10.1093/jamia/ocw118

Holt-Lunstad, J. (2015). Loneliness and social isolation as risk factors for mortality: A meta-analytic review. *Perspectives on Psychological Science, 10*(2), 227-237. https://doi.org/10.1177/1745691614568352

**References 9.7-9.8**

Calder, P. C. (2013). Omega-3 polyunsaturated fatty acids and inflammatory processes: Nutrition or pharmacology?. *British Journal of Clinical Pharmacology, 75*(3), 645-662. https://doi.org/10.1111/j.1365-2125.2012.04374.x

Erickson, K. I., Voss, M. W., Prakash, R. S., Basak, C., Szabo, A., Chaddock, L., ... & Kramer, A. F. (2011). Exercise training increases the size of the hippocampus and improves memory. *Proceedings of the National Academy of Sciences, 108*(7), 3017-3022. https://doi.org/10.1073/pnas.1015950108

Locke, E. A., & Latham, G. P. (2002). Building a practically useful theory of goal setting and task motivation: A 35-year odyssey. *American Psychologist, 57*(9), 705-717. https://doi.org/10.1037/0003-066X.57.9.705

**References Conclusion**

Anderson, E. F., & Taylor, N. F. (2011). The effect of Tai Chi on balance and quality of life in older people: A systematic review and meta-analysis. *Age and Ageing, 40*(2), 242-249. https://doi.org/10.1093/ageing/afq091

Baker, S. (2019). *The Carnivore Diet*. Victory Belt Publishing.

Berry, K. (2020). *Lies My Doctor Told Me: Medical Myths That Can Harm Your Health*. Victory Belt Publishing.

Bosworth, A. (2019). *Anyway You Can: Doctor Bosworth Shares Her Mom's Cancer Journey*. BozMD.

Erickson, K. I., Voss, M. W., Prakash, R. S., Basak, C., Szabo, A., Chaddock, L., ... & Kramer, A. F. (2011). Exercise training increases the size of the hippocampus and improves memory. *Proceedings of the National Academy of Sciences, 108*(7), 3017-3022. https://doi.org/10.1073/pnas.1015950108

Hirshkowitz, M., Whiton, K., Albert, S. M., Alessi, C., Bruni, O., DonCarlos, L., ... & Adams Hillard, P. J. (2015). National Sleep Foundation's sleep time duration recommendations: Methodology and results summary. *Sleep Health, 1*(1), 40-43. https://doi.org/10.1016/j.sleh.2014.12.010

Kabat-Zinn, J. (2003). *Mindfulness-based stress reduction (MBSR)*. Constructivism in the Human Sciences, *8*(2), 73-107.

Taylor, D., Cable, N. T., Faulkner, G., Hillsdon, M., Narici, M., & Van Der Bij, A. K. (2004). Physical activity and older adults: a review of health benefits and the effectiveness of interventions. *Journal of Sports Sciences, 22*(8), 703-725. https://doi.org/10.1080/02640410410001712421

www.ingramcontent.com/pod-product-compliance
Lightning Source LLC
Chambersburg PA
CBHW020543030426
42337CB00013B/964